MW01483515

Beautiful, COURAGEOUS *You*

A Journey of Healing SPIRIT, SOUL and BODY from Depression

LAURALEE BERRILL

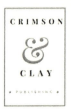

ISBN: 9780646966205 (pbk)
Also available as an ebook:
ISBN: 9780646968827 (ebk)

The stories, suggestions and opinions of the author are her personal views only.The
information and solutions offered in this book are intended to serve as non-medical
guidelines for managing depression: body soul and spirit. Please discuss specific symptoms
and medical conditions with your doctor.

FOREWORD

to Beautiful Courageous You

I first met Lauralee while the pangs of sorrow still raged in her soul. No one should have to endure the pain thrust on her and her family, certainly not the multiplied events of loss and grief.

But she was battling then, seeking to find her way into the light of God's grace and affection that was already dawning in her heart. It would still take her awhile, but I knew then that she was well on the way to recovery and freedom. It's what our God does. I don't believe him to be the cause of our tragedies, but the redeemer in our stories able to take the world's worst pain and work great healing and freedom out of them that leaves us astounded and grateful that he is bigger than any calamity life can throw at us.

This is her story, both of the tragedies that took her to the depths of depression and her ascent back into the light. It is a compelling story, honestly and warmly told, that will encourage and enlighten anyone who has traversed the unendurable.

In the end, Lauralee learned how to let Jesus embrace her in the pain and then teach her how to dance her way out of tragedy into triumph. Depression didn't get to win. Anxiety wouldn't define her future. Now her heart is to help others sort through similar tragedies in their own life and encourage others to know that grief and loss doesn't have to define you. There is a triumph possible in every tragedy and it is worth fighting for no matter how long it takes.

Though you'll find in these pages the honest insights and encouragements of one whose been down this road, keep in mind that Jesus has an infinite number of ways to meet us and set us free. Don't think your answers will come in doing everything that Lauralee did, but in finding the Father Lauralee found. Her counsel in that regard can help open your heart and soul to him, but don't think he will do it in you quite the same way. Our God loves us all and has an infinite number of ways to connect with your heart and lead you into his peace and joy.

You have no idea how hard it is to tell such an honest story as Lauralee has done. She doesn't run from the pain, but embraces God in her grief and despair and discovers that he has the power to lead her out. As you enter into her story, open your heart to the God who invites you into his rest as well, who will comfort your broken heart and mend it with his tender care. No matter how tragic your past, God has a hope and a future for you, too.

And I pray you will find his presence overwhelming your pain, his courage overrunning your fears, and his love warming your heart so that you know you are his beloved child.

Wayne Jacobsen, author of *He Loves Me,* and Co-author of *The Shack.*

DEDICATION

To Jesus Christ

My Lord and Saviour, my source of inspiration and strength.

To my husband, Lee

My ever-present loving support, you are an outstanding example of a Godly husband and father. Thank you for reminding me of my beauty and courage almost daily.

To my children

Rhoni-lee, Jaeya, you are my absolute joy and a blessing to be treasured. Jessica, Jasmine and Connor, my precious angels who are safe in the arms of a Perfect Heavenly Father.

To my family and friends

There are too many to mention. Thank you for your prayers, encouragement and support, without which I might never have written this book.

To my 'review' team.

I take a bow (or a curtsey) to you for honouring my work. Thank you for taking time to assist with the refining process and helping it to become the beautiful expression of hope that I have had in my heart for so long.

To my creative team.

Assisi, I am so honoured to work with such giftedness. Thank you for summoning me into a deeper understanding of learning how to take images from the canvas of my mind and paint them with words. Deborah, you have created a masterpiece; a brand that speaks of love, hope and peace. Your creative ability is astounding. Thank you for making sense of what Beautiful, Courageous You 'looks like.'

CONTENTS

PREFACE ix
About the Cover.. ix

AUTHOR'S NOTE... xi
Healing on the Horizon.. xi

INTRODUCTION xvii
Life is a Story Book xvii
Content, Whatever the Circumstance xix

PART ONE: A SEASON OF SORROW 1
Chapter 1   Apprehended by a Spiritual Force.................... 7
Chapter 2   The Beckoning of God...................................16
Chapter 3   The Refiner's Fire 20
Chapter 4   A Gethsemane Moment................................ 27
Chapter 5   Affliction Eclipsed by Glory 37
Chapter 6   I Am Your Redeemer 41
Chapter 7   Deep Cries Out to Deep................................ 45
Chapter 8   Natural Law 56

PART TWO: HEALING FOR YOUR SOUL
            (MIND, WILL & EMOTIONS) 59
Chapter 9   Change Your Mind, Change Your Life............. 63
Chapter 10   Operation; Free Will 69
Chapter 11   Emotions ... Causing a Commotion................. 75
Chapter 12   Realistic Expectations.................................. 77

PART THREE: HEALING FOR THE BODY.................... 79

Chapter 13   Depression in a Clinical Sense............ 84
Chapter 14   Pathway to Depression......................... 86
Chapter 15   How Exercise Can Help Develop a
             Healthy Mind....................................... 91
Chapter 16   Nutrition for a Healthy Mind 102
Chapter 17   Serotonin Deficiency............................ 108
Chapter 18   Blood Sugar Balance 114
Chapter 19   Medical Approach................................ 117
Chapter 20   Natural Therapies 119

PART FOUR: HEALING FOR THE SPIRIT.................... 129

Chapter 21   Doubt Your Doubt and Believe Your Belief.. 131
Chapter 22   The Journey through Doubt and into Faith... 135
Chapter 23   Living in the Light of Truth................ 140
Chapter 24   A Heavenly Perspective 146
Chapter 25   Past Experiences Shape Your Perspective 151
Chapter 26   Conversation with a Loving Father................ 154
Chapter 27   Praise and Worship............................. 163
Chapter 28   I Forgive Him ... I Forgive Him Not............. 168
Chapter 29   Love on Purpose = Return to Joy 176

PART FIVE: FINAL THOUGHTS..........................179

Chapter 30   Fearfully and Wonderfully Made 181
Chapter 31   Call Back... 183
Chapter 32   Tired of Religion ... I Want a
             Relationship with Jesus 186

**SHARE YOUR STORIES OF BEAUTY
AND COURAGE**.. 189

BIBLIOGRAPHY 191

PREFACE

About the Cover

I wanted to bring hope to the cover page in a graphic sense. For me it was important that the imagery would somehow speak to women, young and old, in an encouraging tone that says "lift up your weary head, let hope arise and be strengthened by the true knowledge that you are beautiful and courageous." The crumpled note being pinned to the wall represents a return to believing the truth about yourself and consequently a return to happiness. Crumpling of the note is symbolic of what we do with our self-belief as life wears us down. As a toddler the words of beauty and courage are written on our hearts and we believe we are the centre of the universe. Doting adults affirm our beauty and we are fearless (except perhaps for the odd monster under the bed.) My five -year-old little girl believes without doubt that she is pretty and perfect in every way. She has no fear of being too fat or too thin and no fear of what other people think. She is free to be a beautiful, courageous little girl. Over the years what we believe about ourselves becomes distorted and fashioned by the influences around us and this is when we "crumple the note," so to speak, and throw it in the wastepaper basket. We gradually lose our five-year-old perspective of how amazing, "fearfully and wonderfully made" we truly are. From an early age seeds of doubt and fear take root in our minds as we become aware of judgement from others, cave into peer pressure, and aspire to be just like the false images of airbrushed models. Doubt and fear grow like relentless weeds, suffocating all that is true about the beautiful, courageous you. May your journey through this book encourage you to go back to the note, which represents your true identity and worth, write out the TRUTH, stick it up on the wall, believe it, and pursue the real you with reckless abandon.

The purple flower is a statice, also known as Sea Lavender; it is a flower of fond memories. It has a very special meaning to me. Many people have a vase of statice somewhere in their home due to its longevity, with a colour so intense that it is simply too hard to throw away. On many occasions I have received a glorious bunch of flowers and long after the other flowers have wilted, the statice continues to display a richly coloured blossom. For me, as long as the flower holds colour, it also holds a fond memory. I am intrigued with how the statice can keep such glorious colour even though the stem and leaves are devoid of life and the plant has long since been uprooted and detached from nourishment. The dried statice on the cover represents how I felt during my journey through depression and grief. My daily struggle with depression made me feel devoid of life, like the dead stem, afraid and ashamed. However, what I have come to realise is that my spirit was alive with vibrancy, colour and hope the whole time, as is the purple flower. On days when I felt too tired to breathe and depression had seemingly won the battle, my spirit never lost hope. The hope remained because I knew I was created in His image; with the promise of everlasting life, born again to choose life, not death.

AUTHOR'S NOTE

Healing on the Horizon

"The most beautiful people we have known are those who have known defeat, known suffering, known struggle, known loss, and have found their way out of the depths. These persons have an appreciation, a sensitivity, and an understanding of life that fills them with compassion, gentleness, and a deep loving concern. Beautiful people do not just happen." Elisabeth Kübler-Ross

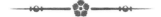

As I start to write this book I feel overwhelmed with where to begin. The desire to write about my journey through grief, depression and anxiety has been birthed from a heart filled with compassion for women who are travelling this long dark road. It is my belief also that nothing is wasted. The years of heartbreak, trauma and terror throughout my life's journey thus far, have given me the gift of perspective and taught me many valuable lessons along the way. Allow this knowledge and wisdom to take you on a journey from *undergoing to overcoming* the battles you may be facing. It is my wish that within these pages you find solace and comfort, and a deep knowing that in your darkest hour there is a reservoir of hope.

Much as in each day the darkest hour is just before the dawn, my prayer for you is that this moment in time is the breaking of your dawn. As you read the chapters of this book may your days begin to brighten. Should darkness relentlessly cloud your mind I would encourage you to read on, and as you do, I believe hope will rise up in you and splinters of sunlight will begin to filter through that dark, cloudy canopy.

Suffering and tragedy are a part of life but what we do with the situations life throws at us makes all the difference to our outcome. Some people shrink back or fall apart when difficulties arise but in the midst of adversity it is important to keep going forward, no matter how difficult the progress seems. In my writing I have shared the key areas that made a difference to my outcome, and quite literally, the outcome was either life or death.

My personal thoughts on the subject of depression, from a healed position are as follows. Depression is seldom discussed openly; it is a taboo subject and one that is not fully understood. When brought up in conversation it is often quickly shelved with a "snap out of it" response. However, I believe there is great purpose in depression, a purpose that acts as a signal to a deeper problem. Depression is more than just a low mood. From time to time we all feel sad, moody or just flat. In depression, these feelings are experienced more intensely, more frequently and most often without reason. Daily function is difficult; just to complete simple everyday tasks is a challenge. Activities that once brought joy become a thing of the past as every breath is burdensome and every thought, deed or action is preceded with the phrase "what's the point?" Symptoms of depression are to be observed as the tip of an iceberg, with the cause for depression hidden deep beneath the surface.

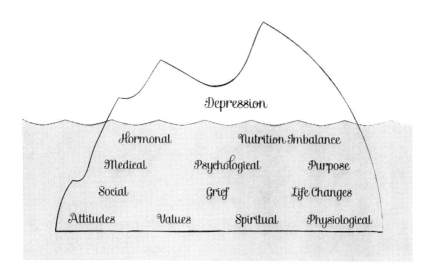

With this in mind, we cannot simply treat the symptoms without exploring the root cause of the depression.

The concept of depression as an iceberg underscores the importance of addressing the deeper issues in three key areas; the spirit, the soul and the body, each of which requires attention in order to be completely healed.

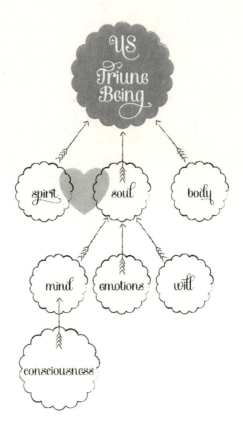

In my experience, depression requires healing on all levels. God has created us as triune beings, we are spirit, which has a soul and lives in a body. I could not simply address the physical aspect by taking medication and hope to get on with life. In like manner *just* seeking good counselling, *just* receiving prayer or *just* exercising daily was not the answer. The journey for healing can become quite overwhelming so I suggest you start small … but at least start! Do something today that will nourish your spirit, soul and body. Get out for a walk, shoulders back and head held high (healing for the body). Chat to God along the way, tell Him all your cares (healing for the spirit) and stop to notice the song of a bird or the beauty of a flower unfolding (healing for the soul). When you lay your head down tonight quiet your mind, turn your heart towards God and thank Him for the journey ... this journey called "life."

I begin the first chapter by sharing my life's journey. I believe the information here will lay the foundations for the building of hope in your own life. In following chapters I write from my experience in nutrition and exercise science and feel that my clinical education supports the suggestions I put forth. But who better to understand grief and depression than someone who has been in the depth of despair? My hope is that as you traverse my personal journey you will consider me "qualified" and therefore allow me the opportunity to offer comfort and hope into your life.

After the foundation has been laid in the first section, the following chapters usher you into a journey of healing for the spirit, soul and body. Together, we will discover what is not working for you and what potentially hinders your attainment of freedom from depression. Life has been a challenge for me, to say the least. What have I done with these challenges? I have overcome them, and my outcome is: inner peace, joy and LIFE!

Come with me on this journey. I don't promise it will be easy or painless. You will be challenged to change many aspects of your life. Change takes courage and can be uncomfortable. It is up to you what you do with life's obstacles. In like manner, it is entirely your decision whether or not you take action and respond to what you read. The choice is yours: to either see yourself defeated and stay the same, or to rise up and take steps towards the Beautiful, Courageous You that you were created to be.

INTRODUCTION

Life is a Story Book

*"The prettiest smiles hide the deepest secrets. The prettiest
eyes have cried the most tears and the kindest hearts have felt
the most pain." Author unknown*

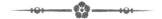

I was born in a small city of South East Queensland, Australia and
am the last of eight children, six girls and two boys, one of which is
my twin brother. Growing up in a big family has it's challenges, as I
am sure does growing up in a small family, but for the most part my
family life was great. My father was a man of solid integrity, gentle
and humble, with an extravagant love for his children.

By the time I was a toddler Dad was completely blind, then in
his later years he was diagnosed with Type 1 Diabetes. I recall us
children having to learn how to give him an insulin injection by first
practising on an orange. He was very brave! Despite his physical
afflictions, my father always had time for his children and always
offered words of comfort and hope when our world was "falling
apart." My dear father passed away at 74 years of age and I long for

the day when I see him again, a day when he is pain free, his sight is restored and I never have to say goodbye again.

My mum has always been a *take life by the throat* kind of woman. Eccentric, smart and witty; she will need several lifetimes to achieve all that she desires to do, and that is what keeps her going. I admire this in my mother. I believe she has inspired all of us children as individuals to be courageous and believe in who we are, never to feel the need to follow the crowd. According to my older brothers and sisters we didn't have a very "normal" childhood, but what is "normal" anyway?

Memories of my childhood come to me as quite simple and enjoyable up until the earliest memory of emotional pain. I recall my early school years as a frightened, lonely little girl; this was when my spirit began to break.

Children can be so nasty. They said I was a dropout and I believed them. They said I was ugly and I believed them. They said I was not loveable … and I believed them. My twin brother was, and still is, the brainy guy in a group. As a twin to the smartest kid in the class I felt shadowed by his achievements, a bar set so high that anything I might achieve wouldn't even come close to the accolades he would receive, so I decided, "why bother!" And this "why bother" attitude earnt me the status of never-good-enough, here I was, a little girl of eight years old, and by grade three my school social status was class dropkick - mercilessly judged by my peers as never amounting to much good at all. School was difficult for me from the beginning. I was absent more days than present and therefore I didn't fit in with the cool kids. In fact, I was a total misfit from the beginning. Truthfully, I despised school. I have always loved learning, but the daily emotional abuse was beyond my level of resilience.

I had little resilience and I recall feeling anxious about leaving home for school every day in fear that my father might pass away while I was gone. In an effort to soothe the anxiety my mother would place a drop of her perfume on a handkerchief and then pin it inside my shirt. To this day, I remember the sense of calm that would come over me with mum's fragrance lingering on throughout the day. School years passed and my father grew more unwell, living on until I was 19 years old.

Content, Whatever the Circumstance

Much has happened since completing school. Like all of us, I have had my share of the good, the bad and the ugly. It has only been in the past few years I have realised that without the negative side of life, we might have difficulty appreciating the positive aspects of our journey.

There is nothing I love more than to sit out on the deck at home on a beautiful spring morning, sipping on a mug of freshly made chai tea. I seldom have time to sit on the deck, much less an opportunity to sit out there on a beautiful day, but when I do get the chance it is bliss. Why such bliss from something so simple? I call it the gift of perspective, an opportunity to view the simple things in life as the most precious.

What an amazing gift perspective is; a gift that comes from the tough times, a gift that takes you above your circumstances and gently reminds you of all the blessings in your life. With the gift of perspective we can see past the discouragement which often follows on the heels of a negative experience, and cherish the small moments, the moments that most often cannot be put into words. The butterfly kisses from my children never fail to warm my heart and refresh my perspective.

Often times when I begin to get caught up with thoughts of "why me?" and lose perspective. I am reminded of my blind father and his ability to press on and persevere in spite of his afflictions. I have wonderful eyesight, what a great blessing! Helen Keller overcame the adversity of losing sight and hearing at age two. Although faced with unthinkable circumstances, Keller counted each day as blessed. She once said, "The best and most beautiful things in the world cannot be seen or even touched - they must be felt with the heart" (afb.org).

When we read what the apostle Paul wrote in the book of Philippians it becomes clear that our perspective on life will determine our level of contentment. Paul wrote from a jail cell;

> "I'm glad in God, far happier than you would ever guess—happy that you're again showing such strong concern for me. Not that you ever quit praying and thinking about me. You just had no chance to show it. Actually, I don't have a sense of needing anything personally. I've learned by now to be quite content whatever my circumstances. I'm just as happy with little as with much, with much as with little. I've found the recipe for being happy whether full or hungry, hands full or hands empty. Whatever I have, wherever I am, I can make it through anything in the One who makes me who I am" *Philippians 4:12, MSG.*

It is so easy to get stuck in the *why me?* trap, believe me I know. In recent years, *why me?* has been the mantra of my life; that was until I realized, "Hey, why not me?" When we develop the ability to look at the bad and the ugly from a new position we can embrace life as a journey of valleys and mountaintops, all of which God draws a line of purpose through. If we have never experienced grief, a broken heart, despair and so on, how then could anyone have an understanding of what another person is going through?

Nick Vujicic was born without arms and legs. I am inspired by his enduring love to see others find hope. He understands pain, rejection, fear and despair and is, therefore, qualified to offer hope.

Nick never received the miracle he'd hoped for, but he believes his life without limbs is far more purposeful. According to Nick, "If God doesn't give you a miracle, He will make you a miracle for someone else."

What is it that draws people to be inspired and encouraged by the Helen Keller's and Nick Vujicic's of our world? I believe there is an invisible bridge, a bridge of brokenness from one person's heart that joins to another's, a heart that understands your suffering and can relate to your pain. A heart filled with compassion will be a heart that offers hope.

Writing about my personal journey through the battles of life is my bridge, if you will, a bridge from my heart to yours. I offer you a heart of transparency, a heart that understands your pain, a heart that is filled with hope for you. The heartache of burying my three babies has at times caused me to doubt God and His goodness, but I have come to realise that He is good and trustworthy. God didn't give me my miracle; He has given me instead a depth of compassion and understanding that I otherwise would not have had if things had turned out differently. In some profound way God has worked all things together for my good. My life (and yours) is His story. I choose, day by day, to let Him write it and rest in the hope that only faith in Him can bring. In the following pages of part one, *A Season of Sorrow*, I will fill in the gaps between when my father died up until this present time. Life is truly a storybook filled with chapters of good and bad. May I encourage you to remember, whatever you are going through at the moment, it is just a chapter … it is not the whole story. As I share my personal journey with you, I do not intend to compare our stories or make light of your suffering in comparison. Rather, I pray that you may be swept up in the arms of Hope and allow the grace of God to carry you through your own season of sorrow.

Part One

A Season of Sorrow

"Comparing your suffering to my suffering is not where Hope is. Hope is in the name of God, Hope is when you compare your suffering to the infinite, immeasurable love of God."
Nick Vujicic

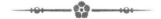

I am blessed with a loving and caring husband, Lee, and we have two beautiful daughters, Rhoni-lee and Jaeya. Some women go through life with their family planning all worked out, confidently assuming all will go according to our 'family planning blueprint.' We plan firstly, to fall pregnant, but secondly, to have a live healthy baby. Some of us may approach having a family as "consumers," with an attitude of, "this is what I want, and this is when I want it!"

I was one of those "well God, I'd like to start a family when I turn 30. I'll have two children thanks. Oh gender? Hmm ... you choose – thanks amen!" Many friends of mine, Christian and non-Christian alike, have experienced frustration and heartache when confronted with difficulty in falling pregnant or have experienced the unthinkable tragedy of a stillborn baby. Personally, I had no problem with conception, maybe it was my genetics? At last count, between my seven siblings and me, we have 33 children! Praise God, Lee and I had no problems with starting a family and I am convinced that as tough as life may get there is no greater joy than knowing we have two little girls to share this life with.

Sadly, for many years the joy of being a mum had been stolen from me. I was incapable of enjoying my children as I worked through debilitating grief. The reason for my grief was the loss of three beautiful babies; my little ones that I had to hold for but a short while before Jesus called them home. Waiting for me in Heaven are my twin girls, Jessica (stillborn) and Jasmine (passed away after 12 hours) and my son, Connor (stillborn).

Even as I write their names I feel an ache in my heart and tears begin to well in my eyes, it is an emptiness that will never leave until our reunion in Heaven. As Christians, Lee and I believe the promises of God, we believe in Heaven not as some religious mumbo jumbo but as a reality of what lies ahead. I will see my children again and until that day I know they are safe in the arms of Jesus. We all experience pain and suffering that can seem unreasonable but I am convinced our suffering and testing is not without reason. Although I have many unanswered questions about God and His promises, I know that He is trustworthy and He is good, therefore in spite of my earthly pain and sorrow I will stand firm on the promise made by the apostle Paul; "For our light affliction, which is but for a moment, is working for us a far more exceeding *and* eternal weight of glory" (2 Corinthians 4:17, NKJV). What a glorious day it will be when our earthly pain will cease and God will wipe every tear away.

Becoming a mother, for me, has been bittersweet. The challenge has been to overcome the fear of loss and feel okay to love my children. In some strange, self-protective way of thinking I believed that if

I didn't allow myself to enjoy my baby, to fall in love with her then I would be able to cope better if something was to happen to her. Although I know now that this is not the case, at the time I had no rational thought. In fact my thoughts were consumed by fear and grief.

My first pregnancy was with the twins. After losing my girls I received no grief counselling. I took matters into my own hands and decided I would just get on with life. Needless to say, grief does not just go away and it wasn't until the birth of Rhoni-lee that I began to grieve and so began the struggle between trying to love my new baby and feeling guilty that my twins didn't survive. I needed to try feeling "normal" so I did what new mums are supposed to do and I joined a mother's group.

I love my daughters more than life but that doesn't mean I need to love everything that goes with being a parent. There are days when I feel out of my depth, as if I am still a child myself and here I am with these little people completely dependent on Lee and I for their every need. I recall my first mother's group meeting, all the mums sat around in a circle and shared about themselves and their little bundle. Every woman had a similar story to tell, "This is baby Jack, he's eight weeks old and I just love being his mummy." I like to wear my heart on my sleeve so there would be no pretending when it came my turn to speak. Before I could stop myself I had blubbered out my despair at being a mum "I hate it, I love my baby but I am overwhelmed with anxiety, severely sleep deprived and my entire body aches!"

There it was, my truth about becoming a mother fuelled by an undercurrent of grief. I had no energy for pretense as I wept before a group of women I had just met. How I yearned for someone, just one person, to be "real" and reflect my feelings. Then it happened. My blatant honesty, it seemed, was the catalyst needed to give the other women a safe place to take their masks off also. One by one they began to share with honesty. Although no one mentioned losing a child, it was a comfort to hear their stories of struggle around being a perfect mum and at the very least enjoying the role of 'mum'. As every woman openly shared with honesty that they too have bad days a sense of unity filled the room. No longer was I feeling like a failure and torturing myself with guilty thoughts like "I should be so happy, I have a healthy baby … I am ungrateful and pathetic as a mum." The act of mums just being real was able to calm my fearful heart. Imagine, if just for a moment, that we could all live our lives from a place of being real.

The freedom I experienced in that mother's group gave me a snapshot of how I wanted to live my life therein … no more pretending, no more masks, just the real me. I cannot count the number of women who have been inspired by me being the *Lauralee* God created me to be. There is something refreshing about a woman that lives life free from the fear of judgement and it is from this place I wish to share my journey of life with you.

There's so much liberty in being free to be yourself
without any judgement from others.

Long before I met my husband I lived a different life. In my late teens and early twenties I went looking for love and fell for a bodybuilding, footballer named Jake (not his real name.) At this stage in life a relationship with God was completely non-existent. While growing up I had been in and out of church and I knew and respected all the "thou shall not's." By the time I reached 18 years old however I had decided a little compromise wouldn't hurt, so … I did!

My personal commitment to God and myself was that I would save my virginity until I was married; this commitment wasn't strong enough though and as my relationship with Jake developed, so too did the pressure to sleep with him. I gave him my most precious gift, my virginity, a gift from God planned for my husband. If there is one thing in this life that I regret the most it is that I did not save myself for my wonderful husband. I realise now that God does not put all His commandments in place to deprive us from having a good time, but rather they are in place so as we do not hurt one another. Having given my virginity to Jake, I was determined to make the relationship work. For three years I endured a very unhealthy relationship as I continued to cling to the hope that things would improve. Being naïve I believed I must stay with him or I would probably be single forever; who would want me after having been with another man?

My father died during the third year of our relationship. Grieving and lonely, I desperately wanted to be loved and comforted, so I worked all the harder to make Jake happy. We moved further north from my hometown for Jake to get work with my brother, thinking this would keep him happy. I reluctantly left my mum and sisters behind. In desperation to keep Jake happy and maintain the relationship my thoughts took a twisted turn and I went off the contraceptive pill. Within a few months I was pregnant with twins. The pregnancy was something to look forward to, a ray of sunshine in my grey, lonely world. Nothing else in life had much to offer and as I moved through the grief of my father's death the thought of having two little bundles to hold brought a new sense of hope into my life. Surely now Jake would love me, cherish me and even want to marry me, perhaps?

My excitement about the pregnancy soon diminished, along with the hope of being loved and cherished. Jake was not at all impressed with the news of a pregnancy, let alone having twins. As my pregnancy progressed he became more and more distant as the idea of becoming a father became a reality, especially when my tummy started to take form of a pregnant woman. Threatened with a feeling of being trapped Jake disengaged from his relationship with me. Late one evening, at week 27 of the pregnancy, I felt a few strange cramps. Jake had not come home yet so my mind began to race with suspicions of where he might be or who he might be with, what if I was in pre-term labour? Have you ever had one of those days when you wake up feeling all is well in your world, and by the end of the day your life is forever changed? Throughout our relationship I remained faithful, true and kind, so to fathom that I could be hurt by someone that was supposed to love me was beyond my comprehension. My thoughts were racing and as I felt my stomach tighten, I knew this was the beginning of labour. I recall thinking "Do I scream, cry … what? Even if I do cry who will care? If I was to scream who would hear me?" Nervously, I picked up the phone and dialed 000 and within minutes the ambulance arrived. The contractions became more intense and frequent; I was in labour. The ambulance officers urgently prepared to take me into hospital, however, just as we were ready to leave, Jake came home. I had no energy to cry or scream, no energy to fight. What was happening was very surreal and I needed to stay focused on my babies and their survival, so I left in the ambulance - alone. Jake didn't follow the ambulance as he had promised. What he did and where he went I do not know. Upon arrival at the hospital I received an intravenous drip of a drug designed to stop pre-term labour and the contractions ceased; it was in that moment that the reality of giving birth at 27 weeks gripped my soul.

Chapter 1

Apprehended by a Spiritual Force

Alone and overwhelmed with fear, I found myself calling on God, my God, the God I had abandoned, the God I didn't need. The whole time I had been trying to do life my way, He was there, waiting for me to come running back into His arms. All my effort and strength was gone; all I had left was to surrender to the hope that I once knew.

Hope in God was buried deep within my spirit. Early years of Sunday school had planted seeds of hope that somehow, someway there was a purposeful meaning to my life. As I turned my thoughts back to God, I cried out to the unseen. In some way I knew He was in the room with me as a weighty peace swept over my being. My broken heart carried a pain so deep that I could hardly breathe. Still in grief from my father's death and in denial of a failing relationship with Jake, I lay waiting, hoping for a miracle … the survival of my twin babies.

I recall that night as the moment when my hurt collided with the healing power of Jesus.

7

I recall that night as the moment when my hurt collided with the healing power of Jesus. I felt simultaneously weak but strong. The apostle Paul tells of the strength he found in Christ: "It was a case of Christ's strength moving in on my weakness. Now I take limitations in stride, and with good cheer, these limitations that cut me down to size—abuse, accidents, opposition, bad breaks. I just let Christ take over! And so the weaker I get, the stronger I become" (2 Corinthians 12:7–10 MSG).

Letting Christ take over is hard for most of us. For me, there was no other choice; I had reached rock bottom with no other option but to surrender my will to His. In a sorrowful situation, we often shout accusations at God and then turn and walk away. I have learned from my past not to curse God and then turn away, but instead to stop and listen, listen for the still, small voice of a loving heavenly Father.

Amid the calamity of the monitor strapped around my stomach, an intravenous drip, and hourly observations by the nurse, I managed to drift into a peaceful sleep and experienced a kind of peace that truly surpassed my understanding. I awoke early to the gentle nudge of the obstetrician on duty. Before I could clear the sleep from my eyes he began, "Good morning, we are making plans for you to be taken to a larger hospital that specializes in preterm labor. It is the safest place to be should your twins decide to come early."

Within the hour, I was in the ambulance and being taken to another hospital two hours away. I was alone and uncertain of how the following days would unfold. The long drive in the ambulance ushered in the opportunity for my thoughts to race, and before long, my peace had turned to dread. On arrival, I was taken for an ultrasound to check on the twins. A cold, stone-faced radiologist performed the ultrasound without speaking a word to me. All I recall is thinking, *God, where are you in all this? This is all my fault and is my punishment for turning away from you.* Why would He want to answer my prayers? I was convinced that God was angry with me.

Finally, the radiologist broke his silence. "We can't do anything for you. One baby is very sick and will possibly die in the next couple of days. Then the other will have a chance of survival. You need to be taken to a large hospital in the city." His words were like missiles, flying off his tongue straight into my heart. No warmth or empathy; just very matter-of-fact. The hours went by very slowly that day. As I lay and waited for the next report on when and how I would be leaving, the same incomprehensible peace washed over me. Like a pendulum, my emotions swung from extreme fear to a deep sense of knowing that despite the final outcome, all would be well.

The hospital decided to keep me in overnight for observation. A nurse explained that there was no point in the expense of flying me to the city hospital if the twins were likely to pass away overnight. In spite of their "prediction," morning came around, and I was still in one piece. Feeling scared and alone, I had managed to get a phone call to my mum. My mother was a six-hour drive away, so I was unaware of her mercy dash to see me, but when she heard of my situation, she dropped everything to get to my side as soon as possible.

Doctors and nurses crowded my room, openly discussing what to do with me. I felt invisible and without a voice. Without hesitation, the group decided to immediately fly me in an aerial ambulance to the city. Some hours later my mother arrived at the previous hospital. It would have been just what I needed—a warm hug and tender care—but my flight to the city had left earlier that day. Needless to say, my mother was saddened and upset with the careless lack of communication. I found out later that although the staff were aware of my mother driving to see me, they failed to call and inform her that I had left for Brisbane, which was now a ten-hour drive away.

Without going into too much detail about my stay in the city hospital, I will say the week I spent there was the hardest of my life. The ward accommodated at least thirty beds, some occupied by women who had newborns, others were there with extreme morning sickness, and some were hospitalized to help battle drug addictions while pregnant. I became a number, my bed number. The staff was doing their best to meet all needs, but they were far too busy to give quality personal care. In my case, I had no appetite and was overwhelmed and alone. To make things worse, I was not allowed to stand up because remaining horizontal was recommended to give my babies their best chances of survival.

By the fifth day of my stay in the city, things looked promising for my twins. Surprisingly, both little hearts were still beating strongly. Although this was good news, I found my heart sinking in despair as I grew more and more exhausted and desperate to go home. I needed to be around family. Even in this desperate situation, God knew my need and in a divine setup, one of my sisters happened to be in the area this particular week and was able to visit me in the hospital. She recounts the moment as being quite disturbing as I could only vaguely recall who she was. Seeing my extreme loss of weight and depressed state, my sister suggested to staff that it would be best for me to go home. Arrangements were made for me to leave the following day.

My family made phone calls to Jake and arranged for him to pick me up. To my surprise, he showed up that morning. With no strength to fight, I promised myself that I would save my energy for my babies, not knowing how or when I may start to labor again. I had to remain calm and stay focused on going home to restore my strength. With barely a word uttered, Jake drove me to my hometown where I stayed with my mum for a couple of days.

My confidence that things were going to be okay began to grow as each hour passed. After so much time away, I was ready to go back up north to be home in my own surroundings. My twin brother had moved in to stay for a while, which was perfect timing for me as it offered me the support I needed from family. So home I went. A couple of days passed, and life seemed to have returned to normal. Although I still had relationship issues, I chose to sweep them under the rug until I had some fight in me. All in all, my time in hospital was just a bump in the road. Or so I thought.

On the evening of my second day back at home, I experienced light cramps and strange pressure down below, almost as though I needed to have a bowel movement. So I went to the toilet and began to push from my bowel. What felt like pushing my bottom actually increased pressure in my vagina. I reached down and felt the crown of a baby! In shock I screamed to my brother, "My babies are coming! Call the ambulance!" Details of this moment are vague as the shock immediately took me into a surreal existence. I do not recall whether Jake was home. All I do recall is screaming to my brother and a vague memory of time spent in an ambulance. I was back in hospital again.

I heard talk between the staff of holding off labor again with an intravenous drip, "No!" I cried. "Please let them be born." I had reached a point where I somehow knew my babies were ready to be born and what would happen from that time onward was in God's hands. In agreement with my decision, the staff allowed me to labor naturally. They did, however, use a drug to slow contractions. As it was late evening and no specialist pediatricians were available, it was planned that I give birth at first light the following day. By five a.m., the contractions were intense and close. As the delivery of my babies drew nearer, so, too, did the urgency of every doctor and nurse in the room. My legs were placed in stirrups, and machines were placed on standby for my babies. Scared and alone, I literally went to another place; my body was present, but my spirit was absent. Or perhaps it was at peace; again, a peace that did not make sense. Truly in my darkest hour, fear and physical pain overwhelmed my entire being until that wave of peace, the peace that was beyond comprehension, reminded me "all would be well."

Labour was difficult. I was engulfed with a sad pain, knowing the likelihood of the possible outcomes. My firstborn, Jessica, was alive and beautiful! She let out a cry as the midwife laid her on my tummy and in that moment I was hopeful. Time went by slowly as she lay there, safe in the arms of her mummy, but the cold reality of her being born too early was about to hit me hard. As they cut the umbilical cord, Jessica passed away. Immediately she was taken away and I was being told to push for the delivery of my second born baby girl, Jasmine. She was born and her loud healthy cry put a smile on my face, a perfect baby girl lay in my arms. I held her for a short while before the paediatrician came to take her for observations and then she was placed in an intensive care crib.

Exhausted and in shock I was confused about whether I should be grieving or rejoicing? Once I had taken a hot shower the nurse led me down the corridor to see my little baby girl. So small yet so perfect, and she was mine. She could barely be seen through all the tubes and bandages that covered her tiny body, but I could reach one hand in through the side hole on the crib and I placed my finger in the palm of her hand. Never will I forget that moment. I knew I was a mother as her tiny hand gripped my finger and my heart ached to hold my baby girl. I stayed by her side all day, and by late afternoon, the paediatrician suggested the best possible chance of Jasmine's survival would be if she were flown to the city hospital. I agreed to do whatever they thought best and within thirty minutes my baby was ready to be moved by aerial ambulance to a city that would be a six hour drive away from her mummy. I went back to my room to get changed and gather my few belongings ready to go on the flight with Jasmine, but the Doctor stopped me in my tracks. "It's best you stay here, wait and see after 24 hours if your baby has survived, then make arrangements to come down to the city." Looking back now, I wish I had been more assertive and confident, more determined to stay by my baby's side. It felt unusual and unnatural to let her go without me, but they had me sign "something" and took her anyway. As the crib was wheeled away my heart ached so terribly that I began to faint due to the completely overwhelming situation. Even though I had given birth to two little girls earlier that day I now stood with empty arms.

The nurses sat me in a wheelchair and took me to a quiet room where I could rest and wait for news on Jasmine's progress. Later that evening there was a phone call from the Paediatrician on duty in the city.He spoke with the midwife and reported that Jasmine was having difficulty breathing and was not expected to live through the night. Ten minutes went by and the phone rang again; the midwife walked into my room and at that moment, so did Jake! My eyes fixed on the midwife in anticipation of what the phone call message had been. She introduced herself to Jake, and then her words "I am sorry, your baby has died," immediately numbed my entire body.

I weep heavily at the time of writing this, as the pain of losing a child is something you never recover from, but my hope in the promises of God gives me a deep peace. As teardrops fall to the keyboard, I can almost hear the voice of my Saviour, Jesus Christ as He whispers, "I am with you." At this time of writing and re-living my past pain and sorrow, I find I have more questions than I do answers, questions which will remain unanswered until I meet Jesus face to face. I am encouraged by the following lyrics written by the band MercyMe, as they have captured in a song, the moment we meet Him:

It's the moment when humanity

Is overcome by majesty

When grace is ushered in for good

And all our scars are understood

When mercy takes its rightful place

And all these questions fade away

When out of the weakness we must bow

And hear You say "It's over now." (YouTube)

How I long to hear Him say, "It's over now ... the pain and suffering in this world – over now."

The pain and suffering for me however had just begun. Half an hour earlier, a new mother had moved into the same room and the sound of her newborn baby pierced my heart. She was surrounded by love; a "congratulations" balloon and bunches of fresh flowers filled her bedside table. The love between a mother and baby can be so captivating, and I couldn't help but stare for a moment as she held her baby and kissed and cuddled the precious bundle. Her heart was full. Emptiness within and without was all I could feel. Physically alive but dead inside, I packed my few belongings and left the hospital with empty arms.

To this day, I still am not sure what Jake was thinking or feeling as we did not speak much. My time was spent organizing a funeral for my twin babies. As I wanted them buried near my father, both girls had to be flown to my hometown.. Jessica was flown from my local hospital where she had passed away and Jasmine flown from the city hospital where she had passed away.. This was a very expensive request and one that I could not afford. My sister approached the local Salvation Army for some assistance to help with the costs and by God's grace they agreed to pay the majority. The funeral was organized and within the week of having given birth we were graveside, saying goodbye to two precious little girls. The pain of saying goodbye was immeasurable; as the baby casket was lowered it became surreal, a vivid nightmare from which I would soon awake. My mind joined the present moment just as the minister was finishing the service with a short prayer. I do not recall his words but as he recited the scripture I once again experienced a peace that surpassed understanding. As the feeling washed over me, it brought with it a sense that "all would be well."

Chapter 2

The Beckoning of God

"There is no pit so deep that God's love is not deeper still"
Corrrie Ten Boom

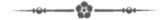

I have come to realize that conflict and crisis often bring about change, and through my crises, God was preparing and strengthening me for some drastic changes that were about to take place in my life.

In the weeks and months that followed the death of my twins, I struggled to make peace with my loss and find the strength to make my relationship with Jake work. Jake went back to his previous ways, however I was changed. In the midst of despair the beckoning of God, calling me towards a better life, continued to surface in my thoughts. About six months after the loss of my babies, in some profound way I experienced courage and hope rising up in my spirit. My grief, pain and sorrow had brought to the surface a strength I never knew I possessed! Day after day, God began to give me a revelation of my true identity; *I deserve better, I am strong, I am beautiful, God has a great plan and purpose for me, it is my right to experience joy ...*

With inexplicable courage I made the decision to sever my relationship with Jake, to break free from the shackles of fear, shame and limiting self-beliefs; all of which our life together was built upon. I recall the day I let Jake know of my intention to leave; I could almost hear his thoughts, "Shouldn't she be depressed, grieving and weak, or at least needy of me?" Don't get me wrong, I experienced all these feelings at once; depressed, grieving and weak, but I also felt hopeful and strong. There was a heated exchange of words hurled at each other Hurtful words? Yes. Did they penetrate my heart? No! I felt God had placed a shield across my chest. May I encourage you, when the bottom falls out of your world, when you are at breaking point and cannot handle anymore, remind yourself of this Truth in the Word of God; " … When the enemy comes in like a flood …" to attack your mind, your marriage, your health " … The Spirit of the Lord will lift up a standard (shield) against him"(Isaiah 59:19, NKJV).

I believe Jesus had responded to my desperate prayers while in the hospital. He had moved in and prepared me for this moment and, as a result, the hurtful words collided with the spirit in me, my healer, my Saviour. How do you respond to such nasty words? I had thought to answer back with insults and fury. Jesus had other plans … plans to respond with truth and grace. I smiled, took a deep breath and the words flowed, "If I can bury my own babies I can live without you. We must part ways, I wish you well." As I spoke those words to my former partner and father of my children, the Holy Spirit breathed in me and gave me strength to forgive him. The feeling of anger and hurt toward him had not changed, but I had made the decision to forgive, to literally release him from his debt. Over the days, months and years that followed, I had to continuously *choose* forgiveness, as I waited on God to change my ill feelings toward Jake. Daily, I had to trust God to heal my heart and to leave it all in His hands by faith, trusting in Him for total restoration.

Choosing forgiveness seems foolish, but it is the right choice to make. Naturally we want to take the path of least resistance, and when we have been terribly hurt the hardest path to choose is the path of forgiveness. In the later chapter of Healing for the Spirit, I write further on the power of forgiveness, but for now be encouraged by the words of Joyce Meyer, who tells us "When we do what we know is right when it is difficult, uncomfortable, or inconvenient, we grow spiritually, and we are strengthened" (Meyer).

Such a tragic loss came to me as a blessing in disguise: the loss of my beautiful little girls gave me courage to make changes in my life so that I might truly "live." I believe God loved me too much to leave me where I was and it was only at my lowest point that I turned toward Him and realized He had a better plan for my life, that His love for me would carry me through the darkness. I don't know what you are facing in your life, but I do know He will bring you through it. Even now I hear an almost audible voice whispering to my heart … "Tell them I love them." Every woman deserves to be valued and nurtured, she is a blessing to be treasured and above all she is truly loved by her Heavenly Father, yes, truly loved more than she can ever imagine.

Much has happened since my separation from Jake. I have grown spiritually and been strengthened by life's challenges. What has changed most significantly though is my *response* to the challenges I face. Life has many lessons to teach if we are a willing student and by God's grace I have learned to respond by trusting in His promises. Despite what my circumstances look like, no matter how hard life gets, He is still in control and He can be trusted. As you read the following poem I pray you also heed the call of Jesus; as you do, may you gain confidence and assurance that He holds you in the palm of His hand … never shall He let you go.

I have been through the valley of weeping, The valley of sorrow and pain, But the "God of all comfort" was with me, At hand to uphold and sustain. As the earth needs the clouds and sunshine, Our souls need both sorrow and joy; So He places us oft in the furnace, The dross from the gold to destroy. When he leads thro' some valley of trouble, His omnipotent hand we trace; For the trials and sorrows He sends us, Are part of His lessons in grace. Oft we shrink from the purging and pruning, Forgetting the Husbandman knows That the deeper the cutting and paring, The richer the cluster grows. Well He knows that affliction is needed; He has a wise purpose in view, And in the dark valley He whispers, "Hereafter Thou'lt know what I do." As we travel thro' life's shadow'd valley, Fresh springs of His love ever rise; Are blessings just sent in disguise. So we'll follow wherever He leadeth, Let the path be dreary or bright; For we've proved that our God can give comfort; Our God can give songs in the night. Streams in the Desert, 239.

Chapter 3

The Refiner's Fire

*He is a refiner's fire, and that makes all the
difference. A refiner's fire does not destroy indiscriminately
like a forest fire. A refiner's fire does not consume completely
like the fire of an incinerator. A refiner's fire refines. It
purifies. It melts down the bar of silver or gold, separates out
the impurities that ruin its value, burns them up, and leaves
the silver and gold intact. He is like a refiner's fire.*
John Piper

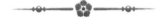

In my devotional reading today it reads; "If you want to know
Christ more, don't be surprised if He takes you aside into a desert
place or a furnace of pain." In the years that followed the death
of my twin girls I went into a desert place, no longer fulfilled by
everyday life. Two years went by and one day I decided to pack my
belongings into my car and drive. I stopped in a city six hours drive
away where I slept in my car for a few nights until I found a room
to let in a lovely Queenslander home. Still in grief and carrying a
heavy depression, I thought that by re-locating things would get
better … surely I didn't need to slow down and deal with "stuff?"

Desperate to get my life back on track and feel purposeful I got very busy *doing life*. Over the next couple of years I worked several jobs in the city, travelled overseas and eventually moved to the Sunshine Coast, where I went to university. One Sunday morning, driving past a local church I felt a Holy Spirit "nudge" to go to church. Apprehensively I took my busy little self into the service. The spirit of God was a tangible presence and within moments I became overwhelmed with a sense of "coming home." Here was the God I had encountered in the hospital, the God that gave me peace in my darkest hour. He had been pursuing me and all the while I'd been keeping myself distracted with busyness. I surrendered my life completely to Him that day, and finally life started to make sense. The peace I had been searching for entered my heart. By God's grace, in a moment of repentance, all of my past transgressions were blotted out, completely erased and I was "born again." To be born again is to receive Jesus Christ as Lord and Saviour of our life and to believe that He died on the cross for the sins of mankind then rose again. As a "born again" believer my past has been forgiven and I am a new creation in Christ. The prophet Isaiah writes, "I, even I, am He who blots out your transgressions for My own sake; and I will not remember your sins". (Isaiah 43:25, NKJV). God has promised to forgive and forget, He gives us a brand new start. Imagine that your life up until now has been a script written by other people's opinions and the circumstances of life. When you give your heart to Christ, He erases the life script you've been carrying for so long and He re-writes it. I discuss this concept in greater detail later in the "Healing for the Spirit" chapter - prayer section of this book.

When you give your heart to Christ, He erases the life script you've been carrying for so long and He re-writes it.

Be cautioned though when you give your heart to Christ and begin to follow Him, life does not magically become a blessed experience where never again will you experience heartache, despair and the general, everyday problems experienced by "non-Christian" folk. Have you ever met a genuine Christian whose life rolls by from one blessing to another? I have met Christians that like to pretend this is how their life is. They have a "church mask" that is worn on a Sunday, to show other churchgoers how holy they are and just how amazing their relationship with God really is (tongue in cheek.) This masquerade they hide behind is what makes many believers feel inadequate in their faith, and by consequence the average believer begins to doubt the love of God. In my experience the religious "church-mask" caused me to doubt how much God really loved me. Most Sundays my inner dialogue would go something like this: "If He really loves me, how come my life is full of calamity and theirs is so perfect? Oh, I really need to pray more, read my Bible more and stop being so grumpy with my kids." In fact, when I was at my lowest point with depression, I would often come away from a conversation with "Ms Super Christian" and feel like I was a stench in the nostrils of God. Oh, if only I knew then what I know now about the love of my Heavenly Father, His Grace, His Goodness and His unconditional love. Jesus says, " … in the world you will have tribulation; but be of good cheer, I have overcome the world". (John 16:33, NKJV). Jesus knew well in advance that this life would be full of trouble, He has not promised that when you believe in Him your life will be trouble-free. He has promised though, that no matter what you face, He will never leave you nor forsake you. Trust me, when I gave my heart to Jesus there were no bolts of lightning tracking through the sky! The devil did not send me a congratulations card and wipe me off his list. What did happen though was that a deep peace moved into my spirit and to this day that peace has been my anchor in the storms. I am almost certain that had I not been anchored in Him throughout the past couple of years, I quite possibly would have ended my life.

God has been good to me; so good to me. I need not look far to count my blessings, and, the greatest blessing in my life has been the day I married my husband, Lee. It was a period of six years before I met the man I was to marry. Before then it was just my dog and I and that was the way I liked it. Having suffered such heartbreak and betrayal with my previous relationship I had determined to date myself, to really get to know who I was and what my dreams and desires were. Basically I needed to heal, not go into another relationship until I was complete. When I gave my heart to Jesus I also made a covenant with Him that I would keep myself pure until the day I married. Some people scoffed and made fun of my decision to save myself and not enter into sexual relations with any man unless it was in a God-blessed marriage. By the time I had met my husband I was complete and carried no further heartbreak. On the other hand, had I been dating men, my guess is I would have been hurt several times over. How Lee and I met and married is a profound and funny story. At the time neither of us was interested in the other, however now, we can't imagine life without one another. Sometimes upon reflection we have a giggle about how we did not plan to be together, but both had surrendered our lives to God and prayed His will be done. Subsequently, His will *was* done!

My husband has been my "Jesus in jeans" since the day we married. He is consistently peaceful, has a genuine love for people, loves God and doesn't just share the message of Christ, but truly *lives* it. His faith inspires me. It never ceases to amaze me how when we "let go and let God" take over our circumstances fall into place, not exactly as we planned, but usually a much better plan than we could ever have imagined. This has been the case with my marriage to Lee. Looking back upon my life I can see where God drew a line of purpose through every situation. Everything I have experienced up until this moment has been purposeful for working towards fulfilling the great plan He has for my life.

After four years of marriage we were ready to start a family and before long I was pregnant with our first daughter, Rhoni-lee. In the early days and months of being a mother my fairy tale-like life was put on hold as the grief of losing my twins came rushing in like flood waters after heavy rain. Up until the birth of Rhoni-lee I was convinced that I had done all the grieving necessary. Grief needs to be worked through, it must be dealt with and I have learned there are no detours through the grieving process. God didn't promise we would never have tough times. He has promised though, that He will be with us through the rough waters. The prophet Isaiah writes, "When you're in over your head, I'll be there with you. When you're in rough waters, you will not go down. When you're between a rock and a hard place, it won't be a dead end - Because I am God, your personal God …" (Isaiah 43:2, MSG). Becoming a mother to Rhoni-lee triggered an almost paralyzing grief in me. As I held my baby … my beautiful, living baby girl, what I had lost in the death of my twin girls became a reality. I was confused. I loved my new baby but began to grieve for the little ones I could not hold. Battle my demons I did … Fear gripped my soul and relentlessly attacked my thoughts day and night. The dread engulfed me, *What if something happens to her? What if I am not a good enough mother? What if they take her away from me because I am not coping?*. Twelve months went by and as my baby girl grew so did my faith, faith that she was going to be okay. I have heard it said that when you become a mother, your heart goes walking around outside of your body the rest of your days. I couldn't agree more; in fact I barely slept for the first twelve months of being a new mother, just in case something happened while I was sleeping. This was crazy and irrational … I know, but this was my way of coping.

Throughout the first two years of Rhoni-lee's life I experienced mountaintops (where life was seemingly perfect) and valleys (where I felt I could not take another breath.) My moods, thoughts and emotions were like a rollercoaster; but all the while God was working out the parts of my life that I had not surrendered to Him. Graciously, sometimes heart wrenchingly, He would lead me through the valleys. These were the days where I would cry to no end, having "picked up the carpet and hauled out everything I'd swept under it." I recall many days of driving down the highway and thinking how easy it would be to drive the car into a light post and end it all, all the pain, all the grief - I would escape. For certainly, I reasoned, Lee and Rhoni-lee would be much better off without me. Sure they might miss me for a while, but long-term the burden of having me around would be lifted and they would carry on. Inasmuch as I was convinced there was no point to my living and felt the desire to end my life, I simply could not turn the steering wheel. Healing came as I allowed the grieving process to take its course. My empty arms were filled with a bundle of joy, a precious little one that was sent to bring to the surface old wounds that were in need of deep healing. Holding my baby girl was also a daily reminder of the gift it is to be a mother, as sadly for many it is not a given and of this I am well aware.

By the time Rhoni-lee was two years old life seemed a blessed journey, almost perfect in fact. Married life with Lee was (and still is) the best thing that ever happened to me. We had a beautiful little blonde-haired toddler and our business was doing well but most importantly, we were living a life of confidence in God. Well, at least we thought we were confident in Him and His love for us. Faith in God is easy when life rolls by from blessing to blessing; however, faith is not faith unless it holds up under great trials. Charles Spurgeon once wrote, "Remember we have no more faith at any time than when we have in the hour of trial. All that will not bear to be tested is mere carnal confidence. Fair-weather faith is no faith" (Spurgeon). The months and years that lay ahead were to be a test of our faith. We were about to experience the furnace of affliction. We would step into the refiner's fire and prove our trust in the unchanging, purifying love of God.

Rhoni-lee was nearing an age where she would be ready for kindergarten and I was ready for another baby. Lee and I were in agreement with having another child and within a couple of months I became pregnant. We were very excited, but also nervous about the possibility of things going wrong. Every morning I would pray and thank God for His hand of protection upon my unborn child. The first six months of my pregnancy went well, extreme morning sickness was all I had to complain about, until late one afternoon when I felt "strange." At first it seemed to be a low blood pressure side effect, a feeling like the life was literally being drained from my body. Lee was busy out in the yard and curiously, I felt that I needed to be near him. So I wandered outside and lay down on the driveway until it got dark. My husband thought it peculiar that I would recline on a concrete driveway at six months pregnant, but he also understood my anxieties about the pregnancy. From his perspective another evening of me worrying about the health of our unborn baby was nothing unusual. Later that night we prayed and put our faith in God to deliver the peace we sought. In this moment His peace swept over me, and the fear was gone. I decided to cast my care upon Him and decided I would wait for my six-month checkup, due in five days, and felt the certainty that everything would be fine. As the days followed I found it difficult to ignore my seemingly lifeless and relaxed stomach. When I am pregnant, my stomach is usually very taut ... "A neat little package," so I'm told, and this felt strangely different.

The day arrived for our six-month check up with the obstetrician. This day also fell on the orientation day of kindergarten and Rhoni-lee was so excited! We were in for a big day; she would find out whether she was going to be a big sister to a boy or girl and she would meet her kindergarten teachers. Her face was radiant with joy.

Chapter 4

A Gethsemane Moment

"Peace is a military move in the Kingdom of God"
Beni Johnson.

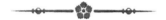

Not long before Jesus was to be arrested and later die on the cross, He prayed in the Garden of Gethsemane, "Father, if it is Your will, take this cup away from Me; nevertheless not My will, but Yours, be done" (Luke 22:42, NKJV). This was His "Gethsemane moment." Deeply distressed, Jesus prayed three times for "this cup" to pass Him by. "Nevertheless," He prayed, in complete surrender to the will of His Father in heaven. Jesus showed us that even those with the strongest of faith can feel weak and overwhelmed in a time of crisis. In our times of deepest sorrow, in the middle of a Gethsemane moment, it's hard to believe that all things will work out for good; in fact, it's hard to believe in much at all. Know this though: it's okay to feel weak and afraid. One of the things we can learn from Jesus in the Garden of Gethsemane is that He understands when we feel overwhelmed and frightened of what lies ahead, Jesus has been there.

The day of our six-month pregnancy appointment is recorded in my mind as a Gethsemane moment, a moment when I was faced with imminent physical and emotional pain; exhausted from deep sorrow, I fell to my knees and cried out "God take this from me." I know we are called to trust Him, but I prayed He would change things so as I didn't have to trust Him. All I could think was, "save me from this nightmare." Author Wayne Jacobsen writes that in every situation we encounter, there are two options in prayer; " 'Father, save me,' or 'Father, glorify your name!' One will lead you to frustration and disillusionment, the other to the greatest wonders in God's heart" (Jacobsen 176).

What began as a day of trusting in a loving Heavenly Father would soon become a day wrought with frustration and disillusion. Our scheduled appointment was at nine am,as we drove to the clinic a strange impending grief washed over me (as if a robe of sadness had been draped across my shoulders). Our Obstetrician, George, was always so warm and caring and he reassured me that I was looking well and healthy, though perhaps a little anxious given my past experience of loss. However "to put my mind at ease," he offered, "Let's have a look at bub shall we?"

Today as I write, my eyes glass over with tears, tears I have not yet allowed to fall. Grief is such a mysteriously long road. I recall the moment both Lee and George could see what I had been feeling – no presence of life in my womb. With tears in his eyes, this caring man turned to me and said, "I am sorry." His words echo through my memory, still fresh enough to produce a river of sadness. Clear memories of what I felt in that moment fail me, the shock and terror of burying another baby gripped me with an iron fist around my throat. I found it both hard to breath and to cry! Lee took Rhonilee into the waiting room so as to shield the heart of our little girl. George next explained that I would be escorted next door to the imaging and x-ray department for a second opinion (to seek confirmation that my baby had died). As we sat waiting to see the radiologist, it became obvious that Rhoni-lee had sensed something was wrong and she turned her attention to me. She started to speak to me of God's love, firmly reassuring me that He was the boss and He was in charge of everything. During the ultrasound she had shown no interest in looking at the screen to see the baby. She was not aware our baby had died. Her attention was focused on me stroking my hair, holding my hand and somehow filling my broken heart with hope. How did she know to comfort me in this manner? To this day, I believe God was speaking to me through my daughter, stroking my hair as a loving father would to reassure a fearful child. The ultrasound confirmed there was no heartbeat and the radiologist offered to tell us the gender of our baby, solemnly he said, "It's a girl, a baby girl."

The ultrasound was over and we were offered two options: to either go into hospital for immediate induction or to leave the process until later in the evening. Despite wanting the nightmare over as soon as possible, I determined in my heart to keep this day as Rhoni-lee's special kindergarten day. We organized to come back that evening and would spend the day as planned. Throughout the day, time seemed to stand still. Lee and I were numb but brave in the face of grief. For me, this day is etched in my mind as the day that I stood "toe to toe with the devil". As all hope evaded me, I believed I had been defeated. In spite of my prayers and belief in God's power to affect miracles, my miracle did not come. Evening set in and I packed my overnight bag for the hospital. Lee's mum, dad and a close friend came to care for Rhoni-lee and she was unusually calm as I explained that her baby sister was not well and we had to let her go back to God. As we drove to the hospital I could not help but question, *Where's the miracle?* My thoughts raced, *God, do you care? Do you listen? Are you even real?*

Disappointment with God turned to doubt and unbelief about His goodness. I tried to believe things would work out for my good, but I could not see how there was possibly any good that would come from such sorrow. As we drew nearer the hospital I recall asking Lee, "Why me? This is not what we had planned, I prayed for a healthy baby ... every day I prayed!" Reality of what we were about to experience hit us both when we walked into the maternity ward, as the cry of newborn babies and abundant joy filled the air.

Here I was again, preparing to give birth to a baby that would not be coming home with me. I knew well the raw pain and grief to be experienced, as we would be leaving the hospital with empty arms. George came into our room, administered the induction medication and gently said, "Now we wait." In silence, Lee and I waited and within the hour my body was induced with a rapid onset of labour pains. George had forewarned the pain would be quite intense; more so than my previous live births. This is because a deceased baby cannot make his way through the birth canal; the body must do all of the work. Four long hours of pain, in and out of the bath, I was on a rollercoaster of emotions. Wanting the whole nightmare to be over, but also not wanting to see my lifeless baby, confusion reigned, and the pain seemed senseless and pointless. Towards the end of labour the urge to push became great, but I was reticent. "I don't want to meet this baby!" I cried. Nature had its way and our baby was born in the birthing pool at approximately one a.m. I did not get to look upon her until a thorough checkup and the cause of death was established. Lee and the midwife helped me out of the water to a nearby bed and as I lay waiting to birth the placenta, I glanced to the side and laid eyes on our baby. At that point everything seemed to be surreal, I felt the same wave of numbness wash over me as I had experienced at the graveside of my twin girls ... perhaps soon I would awake from this nightmare too?

George had spent a few minutes with her and then walked over to Lee and me, with tears in his eyes he sympathized, "I am so sorry." He asked if we were aware of the gender of our baby. I answered, "Yes, it's a baby girl, your colleague already told us during the ultrasound." "In fact," George replied, "You have a son, and he had tied the umbilical cord in a knot, causing foetal asphyxia." A baby boy? We had already named "her." George brought him over to us and showed where his cord was abnormally long and then tied in a knot known as a "true knot." (These cases were rare, so rare he'd never seen this before. Statistics have shown that only one in 2000 deliveries report a true tightened knot, which often causes foetal demise).

By the time we had cuddled with our baby both of us were very tired and in need of rest. We were taken back to the maternity ward where we rested until morning. Overwhelmed with grief, I could not sleep. A light sleeping medication had been preordered to be offered if I could not settle and after taking the sleeping tablet I nodded off and escaped the reality of life for a few hours, so I could be restored and ready to face the day ahead. Morning broke and I recall not wanting to open my eyes. Already, depression was hovering. My baby was gone. The midwife came in to visit and offer some breakfast. I could not eat! I yearned to hold my baby once more. She offered to bring him to us so we could hold him, look at him and then say our goodbyes. While we were waiting Lee had been reading some handouts on the grief and loss of a baby. Somewhere in the pages he found a name for our baby, "Connor" he said, "let's name him Connor?" I agreed, "That's perfect."

Connor was brought to us on a little blue satin cushion, the image of him remains vivid in my mind and will remain until the day I am reunited with him in Heaven, when I will hold him in my arms, feel his warmth, look him in the eyes and call him "my son." He was carefully wrapped in a little blue bunny rug and all I could do was gaze at this little baby, our baby. Lee sobbed from the depths of his being, such pain in every tear that fell. In desperate hope I whispered "Please wake up" but there was no waking, just the cold reality of death. Lee and I were numb in spirit, soul and body. *How do we go on? What now? God, why are you silent?* My thoughts turned to blame, blame for God not intervening. I snarled *You are He that made Heaven and Earth but you could not save my baby? What is that?*

Time passed and it became apparent that we had to let him go. As we handed Connor to the midwife I felt it was important for me to say "You can take my baby now." For in the loss of my twins, Jessica and Jasmine, much of the heartache I still carried was due to the callous way they were taken from me. There was never a moment when, as their mummy, I was able to say goodbye and then let them go. This time it would be different as I foreknew that to begin the grief process it was important that I *gave* my baby to the midwife. As this happened I became overwhelmed with despair. The road ahead was a familiar one for me, but one that I had not travelled with my husband by my side. To this day I am convinced I can endure anything with his support; even now I get a sense of peace and calm when he enters a room to be with me when I am upset or agitated over something.

Lee at all times offers strength for my weakness and in the months that followed this tragedy he became a bastion of strength for me. After time spent with Connor we had to go home and see Rhoni-lee, "She needs me" I cried. We packed our belongings and embarked on a long silent drive home; so empty, so disillusioned, physically and emotionally exhausted. Rhoni-lee, our four-year old, was waiting outside, excited to see us. As we hugged I explained that she was a big sister to a baby boy and he was not well, so God had taken him straight to Heaven. With tears in her eyes she said "That's okay mummy, we'll see him in Heaven." Oh, to have the resilience and "matter of fact" attitude of a child, so faithfully they cope with life's hurdles. Her childlike faith and absolute trust in God made way for her healing to begin immediately, unlike myself, and most "grown-ups." We want the facts, we question "Why me?" Then hurl accusations at God, subsequently journeying through a maze of guilt, doubt, shame and unbelief, until we come full circle back to where we began ... at His feet, completely surrendered. The moment we choose to trust in a loving Father, with the faith of a child, not having all the answers but trusting in the One who does, that is the defining moment in which we receive peace that surpasses understanding, peace which is beyond words. Perhaps that is why Jesus so loved the little children, He took them in His arms and blessed them " ... Let the little children come to Me, and do not forbid them; for of such is the kingdom of heaven" (Matthew 19:14, NKJV).

Childlike faith, it would seem, does not just happen for everyone. Like me, you may have many unanswered questions. "Why didn't God prevent this from happening? Why hasn't He changed this situation?" Sure enough, we have questioned why our path has led us through pain and sorrow, why should we have to suffer this way? After all, Lee and I have honoured and served God in all the ways we know possible, so how come things worked out this way? Did Jesus sit on His hands and let Connor's death top the broken heart charts for Lee and I?

Many times people are perplexed that I choose to glorify God; they have questioned how I can still believe in God, let alone trust in His goodness? They perceive that when I was trusting in Him, He let me down! I have grappled in my mind with these arguments for the past three years. Is God good? Does He love me? Why do bad things happen to good people? In fact, why do bad things happen at all? Finally, I grew tired of trying to figure it all out and made the choice to trust in the Word of God, and as a result my faith has been renewed and I have entered His rest.

I still have painful memories and even present day sorrowful situations, but I am learning to transcend them by actively pursuing God in prayer and through reading scriptures. Proverbs, 3:5-6 implores us to, "Trust in the LORD with all your heart, And lean not on your own understanding. ⁶ In all your ways acknowledge Him, And He shall direct your paths." Day and night I have meditated on this truth. Trusting in the Lord means that rather than blaming Him for what happens, rather than doubting His love for us, we can relax and rest assured, believing that our Heavenly Father has our lives in the palm of His hand.

Mountain high or valley low, I sing out remind my soul, I am Yours I am forever Yours. Brian & Jenn Johnson - "Love Came Down"

Above all else, author Bob Gass implores, "When God doesn't seem to meet your expectations, it's not that He doesn't care; it's that He sees the big picture and He's handling issues you can't even begin to comprehend. So trust Him!" (Gass). I want to encourage you, in faith, to trust in His ways and His wisdom and as you do this He will deepen your peace and increase your courage to face whatever comes your way. He may not keep something from happening, but He can bring you through whatever happens. God has revealed himself through our circumstances as He has brought us through the horrifying loss of another baby.

I believe God, in His wisdom, allows some things to happen where at the time it seems painful and senseless. The very experience that is so grievous and distressing may be to augment your power so as to be of use to others. He sees the big picture of our lives and knows, just like a loving father, what is needed to help us become exactly who we were created to be. I can honestly say you will "grow under the load" as you continue to trust that your Father in Heaven has your best interest at heart as He walks you through the valleys of life and accompanies you to the glorious mountaintops.

Much of my work and leisure time is spent in the outdoors mountain climbing and rock climbing and one thing is for sure, once a mountain top is experienced the mind starts to wonder about the next mountain to be conquered. The mountain climbing experience, for me, is a continual process of growth and pushing to greater challenges and achievements. Likening mountain climbing as a parable for life, Nelson Mandela said: "I have discovered the secret that after climbing a great hill, one finds many more hills to climb. I have taken a moment here to rest, to steal a view of the glorious vista that surrounds me, to look back on the distance I have come. But I can rest only for a moment, for with freedom come responsibilities, and I dare not linger, for my long walk is not yet ended" (YouTube).

Life is both good and bad, mountain top experiences are amazing but most of us spend our lives climbing in and out of the valleys. If all I gave my children were the mountain top experiences there would possibly be no growth, no depth, and minimal compassion to their being. As a loving parent, in wisdom, I allow some freedom with my two children as they experience life and begin to make choices for themselves. At times these choices may take them into a valley, and it's in the valley that I bear witness to great learning and depth in the growth of a beautiful child. Likewise, our Heavenly Father has given us free will, which, at times takes us into the valleys. I am glad for my time spent in the valleys, I am glad for what God in His power did not prevent, for it has given me a depth of compassion and great empathy for those in depression and for the broken-hearted. In His wisdom Jesus takes our pain and makes it something beautiful. As the prophet Isaiah writes, the spirit of the Lord was upon him, "To console those who mourn in Zion, To give them beauty for ashes, The oil of joy for mourning, The garment of praise for the spirit of heaviness ..." (Isaiah 61:3, NKJV).

Today I have beauty in my life, joy which remains immovable and an attitude of praise that leaves the world perplexed. Many times people I meet are completely baffled that I would choose to praise God and glorify Him in every circumstance, not just the circumstances I find acceptable. As you read the following thoughts penned by H. W. Smith, may you be encouraged to praise Him no matter the circumstance, and begin to trust in His tender and wise purposes toward you;

> *See God in everything, and God will calm and colour all that thou dost see! It may be that the circumstances of our sorrows will not be removed, their condition will remain unchanged; but if Christ as Lord and Master of our life, is brought into our grief and gloom, He will compass us about with songs of deliverance. To see HIM, and to be sure that His wisdom cannot err, His power cannot fail, His love can never change; to know that even His direst dealings with us are for our deepest spiritual gain, is to be able to say in the midst of bereavement, sorrow, pain, and loss, "The Lord gave, and the Lord hath taken away; blessed be the name of the Lord"* (Cowman, 277).

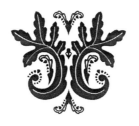

Chapter 5

Affliction Eclipsed by Glory

*"What God can prevent in His power, He permits
in His wisdom" Arthur Burt.*

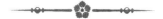

There's no escaping this layer of affliction called "life." There does come a point in time however, when you must decide to either allow the darkness to overtake your life and become a victim of your circumstances, or choose to courageously move against your fears; face every situation and determine to push on, knowing that God is with you. His presence within us is our assurance that we can live in peace. His peace is not just for getting through the tough times, but He has promised us perfect peace and contentment all the days of our lives. Where do we find this peace, this lasting cure for fear? On discovering abiding peace, Bobby Conner writes, "This is the pattern we need to learn: As we turn our inner focus, our will, to Christ and place our affections on Him, adjusting our thoughts to the Word, we will discover abiding peace" (Conner).

Although the scriptures admonish us to keep our minds on that which is Truth, this is easier said than done. In light of losing

Connor, my relationship with God became fractured, to say the least. I knew I was supposed to face up to my fears with faith, but instead of facing up to them, I was overtaken by fear in regards to "everything!" As the days and weeks passed, I slipped into a deep depression. Eventually my faith was all but gone. As I write today, with hindsight, I can see that the situation I thought would swallow me up has become my greatest victory, the truth has set my anxious heart free; for indeed Jesus stated that "We shall know the truth and the truth will set us free" (John 8:32, NKJV). Yet for many months I was anything but free. I lived in fear and anxiety. My greatest fears at the time of losing Connor was that I would slip into depression and also that I would never cope with being pregnant again.

Ponder the life of Job as he allowed fear to rule his thoughts; "Why did I not die at birth?" He lamented. "For the thing I greatly feared has come upon me, and what I dreaded has happened to me. I am not at ease, nor am I quiet; I have no rest, for trouble comes" (Job 3:25-26, NKJV).

In a few short weeks after the death of Connor my thoughts, like Job's, became very dark as grief and sorrow enveloped me. There was no rest, no end in sight. I recall upon opening my eyes one morning thinking, *I wish I were dead.* From that morning on the same thought would harass my mind from the moment my eyelids opened, until the time they closed again each night. Depression had come upon me. The constant battle in my mind had me almost too exhausted to breathe, let alone get out of bed and carry on as usual. There were many days, after I had dropped Rhoni-lee off at kindergarten that I would drive just around the corner pull the car off to the side of the road and weep. In these moments I felt unbearably sad, lost for all sense of purpose and completely exhausted. Tired of being alive, the script in my thoughts on the drive home would play, *Hit the concrete light post, hit this oncoming truck ...* After a month of battling with escalating suicidal thoughts I felt I must speak to

Lee about the torment in my mind, almost as though the enemy attack needed to be exposed and brought into the light to be dealt with. My husband listened with care and concern as I told him of my will to die. Together we cried and hope began to rise up in my spirit as Lee met me where I was. He joined me in that deep, dark place and committed to helping me "climb back out." Many times, just like when rock climbing, I would lose my foothold and fall back into the pit.

On the precipice of denying my faith and completely giving up on ever feeling joy again, I made an appointment to see a psychologist, who "just so happened" to be a Christian lady. At my first appointment, she prayed before and after the session. In a cynical tone, I quipped "good luck with that!" She responded "With what?" "Prayer," I said ... "You really believe prayer works?" "Ah yes," she warmly smiled, "for every client that allows me to pray with them, I have already won the battle for their healing." *Okay, good for you,* I thought to myself. *Maybe this faith thing is a big hoax, or maybe we are like pawns on a chess board that God moves as He pleases, like our lives are some big game for Him to play with.* Yes I was negative, disillusioned and feeling very disappointed with God; if in fact He even existed. However, I pushed on to keep seeing the psychologist and week after week she closed her eyes and prayed for me whilst I rolled my eyes to the ceiling anticipating "Amen" so we could get the session over with.

God began to speak to her as she prayed and one day she suggested my empty arms needed filling; that the desire to love and nurture a baby had begun when I birthed Connor and this desire would not be fulfilled by anything else. I knew this was my basic need, a baby to hold, not to replace Connor, but to be true to my heart's desire. Connor will always be my son and I would never have wanted to replace him with another pregnancy. Deep in my spirit though, I knew the catalyst to my healing would be to face my fears and make the decision to carry another baby. The thought of another pregnancy was frightening. I recall during labour with Connor I cried, "I am never doing this again!" Not because of the physical pain, but the pain of yet another loss would be too great to bear. Perhaps God would redeem what we had lost? Could He really turn our mourning into dancing? Would He eclipse our affliction with His Glory?

Chapter 6

I Am Your Redeemer

Time had passed and three months after birthing Connor, Lee and I were ready to try for another baby. Together we prayed ... and prayed in spite of my doubt that God even existed, let alone listened to our prayers. Somehow in the midst of doubt and unbelief, God was drawing me back toward trusting in His unchanging love. Early one morning, I began to pray "God where are you when life hurts?" I felt Him whisper, "I am with you. When you hurt, I hurt also." I opened my Bible and had faith that God would to speak to me through His word. I prayed for a scripture that I could stand upon, a truth which I could declare in the face of fear.

In this moment, with the somewhat small faith that I had, I heard the Holy Spirit whisper the scripture 2 Timothy 1:7. Uncertain of what the Bible verse was about, I flicked through my Bible to read chapter 1 of 2 Timothy. Here the apostle Paul has written to encourage Timothy in his faith. In verse 7, he writes: "For God has not given us a spirit of fear, but of power and of love and of a sound mind" *NKJV*. In a moment of divine grace, God led me in His word to a truth that I could own, one that I could stand upon and make mine. It was a truth that would strengthen me to once again face my fears of pregnancy. This scripture has been, and still is, the truth I stand upon when all else is falling down around me. In my most recent battles with depression, God's word was all I had to cling to, and in fact, all I needed.

In the midst of my fear and apprehension about going through with another pregnancy, I continued to reflect upon His love and goodness and declared aloud 2 Timothy 1:7. Many days it was all I could do to keep the fear from overwhelming me. As days and weeks passed by, the fear that so loudly shouted for my attention became voiceless as God whispered to my heart "I am your redeemer." I had recognised that Jesus was our Redeemer, but had never really considered what that meant to me personally. Consider for a moment several synonyms for redeem: *to buy back, regain possession of, redeem one's property, free, liberate, rescue, save!* Further, the Strong's Concordance records some of the original meanings of the *name* Redeemer; *kinsman, revenger, avenger, ransom, deliver, purchase, to redeem from slavery, to redeem land, to exact vengeance, to redeem individuals from death* (Blue Letter Bible). Jesus, the Redeemer, is all of these things and has promised to be our Redeemer, yesterday, today and forever.

When God whispered, "I am your redeemer," I believe He was saying "I want to redeem your past hurts, pain and sorrow and I will redeem your dream and desire to have another child." By faith (the very little that I had) I made the decision to try for another baby – God willing. I would do it afraid rather than live with the ever-present ache of empty arms! Lee and I were blessed with another pregnancy only four months after the loss of our baby boy. The time ahead was destined to be a rollercoaster of emotions. As the months went by and the baby started to kick there were many nights I would wake to drink iced water, just to get movement. This was a tip from my midwife, which works well, but the poor baby gets no rest! Truthfully, this pregnancy would be the hardest "walk by faith" I had ever experienced. Weak in faith as I was, I still clung to what hope I had in Jesus and the day I heard Him whisper, "I am your Redeemer."

Throughout the pregnancy my anxiety levels reached a new high. My hormones went crazy and the emotional wreckage and grief were still very raw. I had become overwhelmed with it all and started to feel angry towards God (which I recognise now as part of the grief cycle.) In fact, I was so angry one day that I climbed a nearby mountain, just to get high enough to wave my fist and yell accusations at Him. I figured perhaps He would hear me better from up there! Hormones do crazy things to our rational thought processes. Throw into the mix some anxiety and unresolved grief and you have a fully-fledged, irrational, moody, mad woman!

My relationship with God was bittersweet while I was pregnant, I was bitter at Him for losing my son and then grateful for having been blessed with another baby. I was confused. As the months went by my anger subsided and I decided to pursue peace with God. Peace was afar and elusive. Like a beautiful butterfly settling to rest on an outstretched hand; it stays for but a moment then takes flight again. Peace would settle over me just like that butterfly, just for a moment, and then elude me at the slightest upset. Then I would be left questioning, "Where is God in this then?" Upon reflection of my past experience with fleeting peace, I have come to realise that if I want to have peace that surpasses understanding, I must not seek to understand; I must be content to live with questions and trust that there will be a day when it will all make sense. Nine months went by very slowly, but smoothly. In spite of my anxiety–driven moods, our baby girl, Jaeya, arrived on March thirty 2010. For women who like all the details … My labour was forty-five minutes, no painkillers and a water birth. Lee and I had done it! I had revisited the birthing suite where Satan, the enemy of my soul, had ripped my heart out and taken me into the pit of hell, where grief and fear had gripped my soul and my hopes for another baby were all but gone. Jesus had redeemed to us a beautiful baby girl and together we took back what the enemy had stolen. I held Jaeya in my arms, in awe of the miracle of life and in that moment, I caught a glimpse of Jesus as His presence filled the room with peace, love and joy! Our afflictions had been eclipsed by glory, for indeed God had proven to me that, while He had been silent, never was He absent. God has said "I'll never let you down, never walk off and leave you" (Hebrews 13:5, MSG).

Chapter 7

Deep Cries Out to Deep

"Deep calls unto deep at the noise of Your waterfalls;

All Your waves and billows have gone over me" Psalm 42:7.

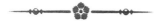

In the scriptures the psalmist poetically alludes to a deer that longs for a refreshing stream and verses 5-7 speak of the sons of Korah struggling with depression, as "deep calls unto deep". I believe this is a cry from the deepest part of our soul, a part that is desperate for intimacy with God, crying out, "I am completely overwhelmed by the trials that have come upon me." In the months ahead of Jaeya's birth I would experience a place where, like the deer with nothing to quench her thirst, I was desperate to believe in God. I longed to experience His heart and all He is, to *drink* of the living water, to go deeper in Him. This longing came from the depths of my soul, completely cast down with nowhere else to go, and the Lord said, "Go deeper." In my experience, going deeper, desiring to know God more intimately, brings your faith under trial, as seen in the story of Job. He was tried, and the latter part of his life was more blessed than his beginning. His faith was deeper, fortified and proven. Perhaps you have cried out, "Jesus, I want to know you, are you real, do you hear my cries?" Don't be surprised if, by way of an answer, He takes you aside into a furnace of fiery trials for a while.

There is great purpose in our suffering, like a refiner of precious silver or gold, the heat is turned up as high as needed for the dross, the impurities of the metal, to float to the surface. To his delight, after he has skimmed the dross from the surface, the refiner can see his reflection and the precious metal is "proven to be real." Jesus takes away the impurities that surface in our furnace of suffering. Although a painful process, the Great refiner knows that this is necessary in order for His precious one to be all that she was created to be ... beyond the refining process. He smiles, for now she reflects His glory. Perfected through trial and suffering, our Lord makes something precious, someone beautiful ... so precious and so beautiful that priceless is your worth!

Beyond the refining process, He smiles, for now she reflects His glory.

"Are not my troubles intended to deepen my character and to robe me in graces I had little of before? I come to my glory through eclipses, tears, death. My ripest fruit grows against the roughest wall. Job's afflictions left him with higher conceptions and lowlier thoughts of himself. "Now," he cried, "my eye seeth thee" (Cowman, 294).

At this time of recall and recording of my "fiery trials" in writing, Jaeya is a cheerful little five-year old. She lights up our world, truly a gift straight from the throne of Heaven. I still have my ups and downs, on occasions I feel as though I am back in the furnace, but the difference these days is that I have a deeper, more intimate relationship with God. I believe, and have learnt, that however hot the furnace may be His hand is on the thermostat and He is always in control. However, this was not the case for the first eighteen months of having Jaeya. During this time a great battle raged in my mind, as the enemy sought to extinguish my hope and my faith in God.

Two months after my daughters' birth, sleep deprivation was building up and I was feeling overwhelmed and weak with the dark thought patterns of depression returning to haunt me. Postnatal depression had set in and unfortunately I was to discover later that this is more common than we recognise. A combination of minimal and interrupted sleep, fluctuating hormones and isolation at home with a new baby can leave our minds open to anxieties and irrational thinking. When we are completely exhausted, we can hear the whispers: "You're never going to amount to much, nobody cares about you, life is going by without you, you're lonely, depressed and useless." These are the thoughts I began to ruminate on. As the weeks went by they became a loud voice getting stronger as my faith grew weaker. I found it hard to eat and hard to sleep; all I could do was cry! Where had my faith gone? How did I get here?

A little while prior to having Jaeya, I had committed to speaking at a women's group on the topic of overcoming grief and depression! How could I go and speak about a topic that I was still battling with? Here I was back in the pit of hell, I had nothing to offer these women! Needless to say, I did have a testimony of endurance through losing three babies and battling depression … apparently I was "qualified" to speak into the lives of other women and offer hope. It was at this speaking engagement that fear and low self-esteem began to take control. I felt I did not belong there for I had not yet arrived at a place of joy. In fact I had gone backwards! During the introduction of their "special guest" (me) I was thinking: *Hypocrite, you cannot speak on how God has healed you from depression and blessed you with Jaeya … you don't really believe that!* In spite of these thoughts, I pressed on. With the faith of a mustard seed, I presented at the event. We laughed, we cried and hope was imparted from my heart to theirs. After the speaking event was over I sat in my car and an almost audible voice entered my mind: *Who do you think you are? Hypocrite!* A panic attack came over me and this marked the beginning of my spiral back into depression.

For the next eighteen months I would go through the motions of being a mother and wife, while every day I fought with the feeling that I could not go on. Upon waking, I would curse the morning sun as I dragged myself into facing another day.

It was a rainy day and I was at my lowest point. I cried all morning, convinced that my life amounted to nothing. No matter how many people told me that life does count, that I had a beautiful family and a great future, nothing could help me "snap out of it." I was depleted; physically, emotionally and spiritually. How did I get here? How do I get out? So scared of thoughts about wanting to end it all, I began to shake. In need of fresh air to clear my head I gently placed Jaeya in her cot. Knowing she was safe, I went to the backyard, fell to my knees in the pouring rain and cried, "God where are you? If you are real, save me from myself, I cannot take anymore!" Twenty minutes went by and still I had heard nothing. I questioned Jesus, my Redeemer. "Why are you sitting on your hands when you could deliver me from this living hell?" There was nothing: no peace, no presence of God - just the heavy rain falling upon my exhausted tear-stained face.

Dragging my sorry self inside, I wrapped a towel around my waist, sat down and picked up my mobile phone. I was desperately in need of someone to talk to. A good friend of ours came to mind. Janet was like a mother to Lee and me, and although we had not spoken for a few years I felt compelled to give her a call. God was at work. Hands trembling, I dialed her number. She answered with a gentle hello and I burst out "Janet, I need help!" I then proceeded to fill her in on the past couple of years and all that had happened. Nearly speechless, Janet offered, "I don't know what to say! But I do go to a prayer group on Thursdays, you should come." I had not been to church for quite a while so I was apprehensive about some religious group get-together ... As I finished the phone call, I felt a glimmer of hope rising in my spirit. If I could just hang on until Thursday, maybe God would show up and heal me?

Many obstacles stood in the way of what would become the beginning of my journey into the very heart of God. Although I was apprehensive right up until the moment of leaving home, when I did arrive at the prayer meeting I discovered that there were many familiar faces from my early church days and I felt a presence in the room in the form of a tangible, thick love. My spirit could sense the presence of God, even if my mind warred against it with accusations of doubt and unbelief. The battle between the soul which consists of the (mind, will and emotions) and the spirit, is fierce. "Your battleground is not the circumstances of your life. The true battleground of the enemy is in your mind, will, and emotions. Keeping your thoughts and heart focused on good things will prevent darkness from overtaking your soul" (Conner).

I have intimately discovered that to have abiding peace we must stay focused on Jesus and His word. The apostle Paul put it perfectly when he wrote:

> "Finally, brethren, whatever things are true, whatever things *are* noble, whatever things *are* just, whatever things *are* pure, whatever things *are* lovely, whatever things *are* of good report, if *there is* any virtue and if *there is* anything praiseworthy—meditate on these things. [9] The things which you learned and received and heard and saw in me, these

do, and the God of peace will be with you" (Philippians 4:8-9, NKJV).

When the war rages in your soul – and indeed it will, as the mind conspires against the spirit, do not run from fear, but instead stand firm in your faith "casting down arguments and every high thing that exalts itself against the knowledge of God, bringing every thought into captivity to the obedience of Christ"(2 Corinthians 10:5, NKJV).

I realised through attending the prayer group that my mind had been given free reign: it was accustomed to running wild and to focusing on fear and anxiety. As we submit to God and resist the devil (our true enemy) the Holy Spirit moves in. However, it is during this time that the mind becomes a battlefield. As we are being renewed to new ways of thinking the enemy will take any opportunity and attempt to steal our peace, hope and joy. In my first moments at the prayer group I stepped into the presence of God and subsequently my mind pushed to the forefront, with thoughts of doubt, unbelief and confusion (all thoughts from the pit of hell). As my spirit was bearing witness to the tangible love in the room, everything within me wanted to run with fear. My mind suggested, *There is no hope for you, this is a cult, if God is real He does not have enough mercy for you.* One of the ladies, Linda, discerned my inward struggle. "You okay honey?" she asked. I burst into tears, "No, I am not okay, I feel like giving up, I don't want to live anymore, I am tired of the struggle of willing myself to live every day and I am not so sure I believe in God anymore!" This experience has shown me that there is no equal to strong, faith-filled women when our boat is sinking (although mine was already in the depths). This faithful woman smiled and responded to my fear with, "That's okay honey, we'll pray for you anyhow."

This was not a time to run in fear, but rather, to stand firm in faith despite being bombarded with thoughts of skepticism, anxiety and confusion. I agreed to receive prayer from the group of women. Now, I have never been what I would label as a "super spiritual" Christian, but for those of you who doubt God wants to baptise you in the Holy Spirit, I suggest you surround yourself with some Jesus loving intercessory women. Get them praying for you and then buckle up! Within seconds of the group beginning to pray for me, I was baptised in the Holy Spirit, speaking in tongues and trembling under the anointing. This was the anointing I had heard about, witnessed happening to others, but never thought it would happen to me! If you have never experienced the anointing, you may be thinking: "Well Lauralee, is it possible you were anxious, disillusioned and in need of a rest?" Truthfully, I questioned what was happening as well. Once the prayer session was over, I cried, "What just happened to me? I feel different, I feel I am healed." God had filled me with an outpouring of the Holy Spirit as I was shaken to the core. Something happened in that moment of prayer, something that makes no sense at all to the human intellect, but I was spirit-filled and could feel the power of God running through my body, followed by peace - perfect, supernatural peace. What was this inexplicable peace? Author, Bobby Conner puts it well, "Nirvana will not be generated by people. It is not obtained through yoga or occult meditation or any other occult practice. True tranquility of the soul, genuine godly peace, is only found in the person of Christ. *He alone is the Prince of Peace*" (Conner).

This was not a once-only experience. God has continued to fill me with His presence and often has given me dreams and visions regarding my life and the lives of others ... I *am* "spirit-filled"! When I returned home after the prayer group I called my sister on the phone and shouted down the receiver, "God is real, I am healed!" I was overflowing with joy. How was it possible to move from a deep depression into being overcome with joy? This is not the result of positive thinking, it is impossible to change a negative thought pattern in the space of a few hours! But, with God, all things are possible. Through the power of prayer I had God's Word, the Truth, spoken into my spirit and this was the beginning of the breaking off a multitude of lies the enemy had been whispering to me. Truth is powerful. The Bible tells us that the Word of God is "living and powerful and sharper than any two-edged sword" (Hebrews 4:12, NKJV). The Word is the greatest weapon of all. When you hear or read the word of God and you know the truth of who you are, then you stand firm, with true determination and resolve that you are more than a conqueror, that you are loved by God. This perseverance leads to breakthrough; without fail. Nick Vujicic understood this when he said: "In life, if you don't know the truth, then you can't be free, because then you'll believe that the lies are the truth. But once we realize that when we read the Word of God and you know the truth of who you are, then I'm not a man without arms and legs. I am a child of God " (Watts).

So why did God move in such a powerful way to bring a miracle healing upon me? I believe He answers the cry of a desperate heart. We must thirst and long for God, surrender our lives to Him completely. For most of us, we only completely surrender as I did once there are no other options. The prayer group was my final attempt to get well. Begin today to truly seek Him with your whole heart, and expect Him to answer your cry for help. If you feel distant from God, I assure you, He is not the one who has moved.

If you feel distant from God, I assure you,
He is not the one who has moved.

The story is told of a young student, who went to his spiritual teacher and asked the question,

"Master, how can I truly find God?" The teacher asked the student to accompany him to a river that ran by the village, and invited him to go into the water. When they got to the middle of the stream, the teacher said, "Please immerse yourself in the water." The student did as he was instructed, whereupon the teacher put his hands on the young man's head and held him under the water. Presently the student began to struggle. The master held him under still.

A moment passed and the student was thrashing and beating the water and air with his arms. Still, the master held him under the water. Finally, the student was released and shot up from the water, lungs aching and gasping for air. The teacher waited for a few moments and then said, "When you desire God as truly as you desired to breathe the air you just breathed - then you shall find God" (Biblecenter.com).

"When you desire God as truly as you desired to breathe the air you just breathed - then you shall find God"

For those who are in the midst of suffering now I say this - God wants to heal you from depression, anxiety, shame, addiction and whatever else holds you captive. He wants you to dream again and dream big! Have a vision for your life that captures your heart and imagination; something so big that you become purpose-driven. For this to happen, you must first confront your captors - your past hurts and habits. Unforgiveness must be dealt with before you can launch out into a new life of complete freedom and joy where you are ready to dream again, to truly live again! Doing this requires courage and plenty of it! Author, Bob Gass writes: "On the heels of every dream there's a demon of doubt. No sooner is your dream conceived than your mind is suddenly filled with all the reasons why it may not work ..."(Gass). Your inner dialogue might go something like this: "receiving prayer does not really work and going to a counsellor would be a waste of time." You perhaps feel that you have been this way for so long now that you are doubtful anything will ever change. You could say that "this is just the way I am." Gass continues, "And there will be folks around you who'll be quick to confirm those fears. In spite of that, you must forge ahead and dream; otherwise you'll spend the rest of your life fulfilling the dreams of others." (Gass). It is time to stand firm and declare that you will not stay this way. Break free from the shackles of fear; God has more for you than you have been settling for.

You've heard it said, "The first step is always the hardest." I found this to be most apparent when faced with my first appointment to see a psychologist, and then again when I had to admit I needed frequent sessions with a counsellor. I was ready to admit my need for help and I believe the Holy Spirit was leading me to deal with past grief and sadness from my childhood.

"Rise up; this matter is in your hands ... take courage and do it" Ezra 10:4, NKJV.

Seeing my need for counselling a good friend,gave me a business card of a Christian Therapist. I attended her practice for as long as I felt I needed support. From my first meeting with this counsellor, my life has been a "new normal." Life has changed from being lived half-heartedly and merely hoping that God was real, to a daily intimate relationship with my Heavenly Father. His love has captured my heart and brought healing and peace into every area of my life. How has this happened? As I mentioned at the beginning of this book, many factors have contributed to my healing. In particular, I recall a session with my therapist where she facilitated an emotional healing technique also known as the "Healing Pool." This concept is a method of emotional healing based on the story of the lame man who waited by the spring fed pool of Bethesda to be placed on its healing waters (John 5:1-9). Using imagery and symbolism, my counsellor used this technique to help me establish what strongly held beliefs I had that did not align with the word of God. This session is clear in my mind as the time when I felt a strange freedom in my thought life, all lies that governed my life (lies of insignificance, that I was not good enough, that I would never measure up, lies of purposeless, that I was not loveable and there was no real purpose to my living) were replaced by truths that Jesus presented to me during my healing pool experience. The most significant change being that the ever-present sadness, which I carried for as long as I can recall, had gone. There is now no amount of untruth that can separate me from God's love. This can only be explained as a God-breathed miracle. You might say, "Can that happen for me? I have never read the Bible, I don't go to church, why would God do that for me?" God is not moved by religious acts and moral uprightness, He's moved by faith. In the words of Jesus: " ... The one who comes to Me I will by no means cast out"(John 6:37, NKJV).

God is not moved by religious acts and moral uprightness, He's moved by faith.

If you are willing, He is waiting for you. If you have never given your heart to Jesus, you might find useful the prayer I have written at the back of this book, simply to ask Him into your heart.

Chapter 8

Natural Law

Besides the spiritual laws, we also have natural laws. As touched on earlier in this book, I believe we cannot address depression and anxiety on just one level. To be completely healed, we must consider ourselves as the triune being that we are. From my past experience as a medical representative for antidepressants and with a background in Health Science, it was obvious to me that there was much more to be done for complete healing. It was for this reason that, alongside frequent prayer and ministry for anxiety and depression, I thoroughly researched what, on a practical level, my physical body required in order to regain health. During my sessions with a psychologist and a professional counsellor, who both operated under God's guidance, it also became apparent that besides the physiological needs, the soul (mind, will and emotions) plays a key role in the healing process. The following chapters are the result of much research, trial, error and simple common sense. Please understand that while I did not personally make use of prescription medicines, I believe medication used in the right context can be a useful resource to assist in the treatment of depression. I made the choice to pursue my healing without the use of medication of any kind for two reasons in particular. Firstly, it was most important for me to continue to breastfeed my baby without drugs in my system. Despite research claims stating that antidepressants are safe to use during breastfeeding, this was personally not a risk I was willing to take. Secondly, I do not believe a drug (of any kind) could have healed my broken heart. There are no detours around grief, we must courageously work through the pain and sorrow; I preferred not to numb my emotions as I found that I needed to "feel to heal".

May I take this opportunity to encourage you to seek professional medical advice before you go off any medication and/or before you choose to take a natural approach towards the treatment of depression. Throughout these past few years, I have had my Medical Practitioner involved every step of the way. He has monitored my general health and ensured that, if at any point I required medical assistance, he was aware of the natural supplements I was taking which could have contraindicated any prescription medication.

The fact that you are still reading thus far into this book is a sure sign that you are willing to take steps towards your healing from depression. It takes courage and lots of it. Firstly to admit that you have depression and anxiety or that you are just not coping with life for any other reason, and secondly, that you would like to do something about it!

My prayer for you is that you have already begun to experience hope through the words of my testimony and that the healing will continue to flourish as you journey through the following chapters. I truly believe with all my heart that as you hold this book in your hands, you have made a declaration to be the overcoming, awesome woman you were destined to be. In spirit I see you "drawing a line in the sand." As you step over that line, you are stepping into the realisation of your true identity. The truth will set you free and day by day you will rise up and behold the Beautiful, Courageous You!

PART TWO

HEALING FOR YOUR SOUL (MIND, WILL & EMOTIONS)

"God has given us a design of hope: we can switch on our brains, renew our minds, change and heal."
Dr. Caroline Leaf

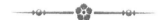

Before we can heal the soul we must first understand what the soul is. I mentioned in the beginning of this book that God has created us as a triune being; we are *spirit*, which has a *soul* and lives in a *body*. In pursuit of healing the soul it is most important to understand that the soul consists of the mind (which includes the conscience,) the will and the emotions. The soul and the spirit are mysteriously tied together and make up what the Scriptures call the "heart."

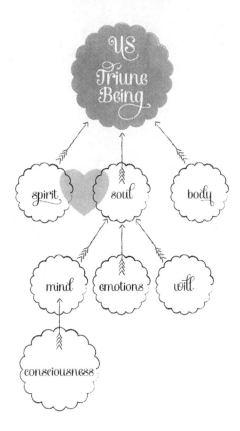

The writer of Proverbs urges: "Keep your heart with all diligence, for out of it *spring* the issues of life" (Proverbs 4:23, NKJV). We see here that our "heart" is central to our will and emotions, Gill's Exposition puts it this way, "for out of it are the issues of life; of natural life: it is the seat of it, from whence all actions of life are derived; it is, as philosophers say, the first that lives, and the last that dies" (Bible Hub).

The verse we just looked at is fairly clear – springs of life flow from a healthy soul. To bring healing to the soul we must watch with all diligence, guarding the heart from all that would cause the spring, the stream of life that proceeds from it, to be sealed up. Failure to guard the heart will leave our spirit and soul vulnerable to fear-based living, where no life flows, a life personified as a "deadman walking," one that carries the burden of a depressed heart.

Failure to guard the heart will leave our spirit
and soul vulnerable to fear-based living.

One of the great mysteries of the unity between body, soul and spirit is how our internal realities affect our external realities. Author, Randy Clark writes on *Healing and a Prosperous Soul*:

> There is an intrinsic connection between the health of a person's soul and his or her overall physical health. While I do not believe we should conclude that every disease is connected to some malady of the soul, I do believe our health is powerfully connected by how we think, what we feel and how we choose to do life. This realm called the *soul* calls the shots more often than we might imagine (Johnson and Clark, 178).

Chapter 9

Change Your Mind, Change Your Life

"In my experience the mind has been my greatest challenge in
overcoming depression, if you can change your mind
you will change your life."

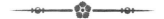

As discussed briefly in the Forgiveness section, chapter twenty-eight, of this book, science has discovered that 87 – 95 percent of current mental, physical and emotional illnesses come from our thought-life. When our thoughts are negative, our mind is in torment, filled with chaos and by consequence, chaos reigns in our bodies. Dr. Caroline Leaf, a cognitive neuroscientist and author explains the link between our thoughts (mind) and the affect they have on our spirit and body. Dr. Leaf asserts that because people cannot see a thought they tend to think of thoughts as harmless. But a thought is real. It occupies mental real estate. As you read these words, have a conversation, listen and think about things, you are building what science call the "magic trees of the mind" so called because the nerve cells in the brain look like trees. Literally, we have these forests of tree branches in our mind, thoughts are not fleeting, they are real, real trees that we build in our brain. Dr. Leaf writes:

As you think, your thoughts are activated, which in turn activates your attitude, because your attitude is all of your thoughts put together and reflects your state of mind. This attitude is reflected in the chemical secretions that are released. Positive attitudes cause the secretion of the correct amount of chemicals, and negative attitudes distort the chemical secretions in a way that disrupts their natural flow. The chemicals are like little cellular signals that translate the information of your thought into a physical reality in your body and mind, creating an emotion. The combination of thoughts, emotions and resulting attitudes, impacts your body in a positive or negative way (18).

Your mind and body are essentially linked, and every thought marks the start of this intricate association whereby our thoughts can create physical changes in our bodies, right down to genetic levels. Research has demonstrated that a negative thought-life can restructure the cell's makeup causing sickness and disease to take hold of the body. In like manner, a positive thought-life will promote healing for the body and mind.

Now we understand the importance of a positive thought-life we have to recognise when a negative thought enters our mind. The mind is a battlefield and our enemy, Satan, wages war on our mind and seeks to defeat us with worry, doubt, fear, anxiety, depression, confusion and negative thoughts that "comes to mind." Joyce Meyer has written a bestseller on this topic, *Battlefield of the Mind*. On the devil's cunning deception she writes: "He begins by bombarding our mind with a cleverly devised pattern of little nagging thoughts, suspicions, doubts, fears, wonderings, reasonings, and theories" (17). Over time the negative thoughts take root in our minds as being the truth, or otherwise known in science as the toxic trees. The biblical term for thoughts that are negative is referred to as a stronghold, "an area in which we are held in bondage (in prison) due to a certain way of thinking" (18).

For example, a daily thought pattern for me when suffering depression would run like this: *Life is not worth living, I am worthless and I will never be happy again.* This train of thought would play over and over in my mind keeping me oppressed, depressed and in bondage, a prisoner held captive by my thoughts. You may be experiencing this battle in your mind as you read the pages of this book, maybe you have strongholds in your mind, scripts you have been playing for years that you're not even sure are yours or even how they got there. Let me encourage you, God is on your side, He will not forsake you. There is a war going on and your mind is the battlefield but here's the thing, as Satan attempts to build strongholds in your mind rest assured, we have all the weapons we need to tear down the strongholds. Strongholds in the mind are, in essence, deceptive lies and false beliefs. The Bible has promised you shall know the truth, and the truth shall make you free (John 8:32). I believe what Jesus was saying is that the truth (God's word) is our primary weapon for tearing down strongholds. Consider it this way, the opposite to a lie is truth, therefore the more time you spend immersed in truth (reading the Bible, hearing Biblical teaching,) the more light of God is shed upon the darkness, and upon the lies in your mind.

Without question, the truth will dispel the darkness. That my friends is the power of God's word! Take a simple example of walking into a dark room, we switch the light on and the dark is gone instantly, light and dark cannot coexist and so it is with truth and a lie. So go ahead "switch some lights on," disempower Satan's ability to influence your thoughts.

Instead of getting overwhelmed with all the work you have to do to correct your thinking may I remind you that in Christ the battle is already won, understand that your identity in Christ is that of an overcomer and *more than* a conqueror. We do not fight *towards* victory; we fight *from* a place of victory. First Corinthians 10:13 promises, "No test or temptation that comes your way is beyond the course of what others have had to face. All you need to remember is that God will never let you down; he'll never let you be pushed past your limit; he'll always be there to help you come through it" (1 Corinthians 10:13, MSG).

Changing your mind and tearing down strongholds is hard work, it takes discipline and is strongly opposed by Satan. In fact, it is impossible to do it on our own but with God, it is possible. Our mind likes to take the driver's seat. Up until you take authority over your thought-life, the mind is convinced it is master. Our thoughts take the path of least resistance until they are opposed with Truth. The truth is, you have been created in the image of God, search your heart where faith abides and live from there. We are wired for love in terms of happiness, peace, joy, excitement and the like. Literally, the neurons in our brain are wired in a positive direction, in a healthy direction. However if we choose to think in a negative direction, make bad choices and hang onto what is negative: anger, abuse, irritation etc., a physical change occurs in the brain; we re-wire the brain in a negative direction and literally build toxic trees. The great news for you and I is that science has discovered that these toxic pathways in the brain can be rewired. Brain imaging is a tangible example of God's teaching on the ability of the mind to be renewed. Science has finally caught up with the Bible. Johannes Kepler, the famous mathematician and astronomer, once said, "Science is simply thinking God's thoughts after him" (56). In other words, God established the laws of neuroscience and then we discovered them.

In the Bible, with wisdom way ahead of science, the apostle Paul writes: "And do not be conformed to this world, but be transformed by the renewing of your mind ..." (Romans 12:2, NKJV). I believe the apostle Paul understood the physiological effect of thinking on that which is negative where he later instructs in the book of Philippians, to *think about what you are thinking about*: "Finally, brethren, whatever things are true, whatever things *are* noble, whatever things *are* just, whatever things *are* pure, whatever things *are* lovely, whatever things *are* of good report, if *there is* any virtue and if *there is* anything praiseworthy—meditate on these things" (4:8, NKJV).

In depression the mind focuses and ruminates on all negative thoughts, past and present. As we approach each day with good intentions to read the Word and pray we can get caught up in thinking that it's all a waste of time, nothing works and "this is just the way I am;" throwing our arms in the air and breathing a big sigh of defeat. In my case I would sit on the floor in a heap and scream at God and then go on ignoring Him for the rest of the day because He had not healed me.

You must, I repeat, *must* press through that which holds you back from using your warfare weapons (prayer, reading the Word, speaking the Word and praising Him). Paul explains it this way; "For though we walk in the flesh, we do not war according to the flesh. For the weapons of our warfare *are* not carnal but mighty in God for pulling down strongholds, casting down arguments and every high thing that exalts itself against the knowledge of God, bringing every thought into captivity to the obedience of Christ ..." (2 Corinthians 10:3-5, NKJV).

Set a purpose in your heart to continue talking to God about how you are feeling or simply praise Him for His promises. As you do this your mind will be renewed, change the things you allow your mind to dwell on and create new trees, re-wire, or as my counsellor once put it "pray, God re-boot me to the manufacturers original default settings." Think about this, if all the thoughts you've had up until this point have not made you feel any better, have another thought. As you pursue God He will eclipse your fears, broaden your horizons, change your perspective and you will have another thought, a thought which comes from His heart and you will begin to see yourself and your circumstances as He does, through eyes of faith, hope and love. Rejoice in this truth – now there's a thought!

Chapter 10

Operation; Free Will

*"God designed us for joy. He created us to have more wealth
in our souls than the greatest billionaire of our day has money
in the bank." Randy Clark*

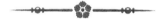

God created us to operate with a free will. You and I have been given the ability to choose what we do and what we don't do. As previously discussed, we have the ability to choose what thoughts we accept or reject and therefore we also have a God-given ability to renew our mind. However, an undisciplined mind allows all manner of negative thoughts to take root and grow. Our negative thoughts and beliefs then become our reality, a life of negative experiences. For example, when I was in depression and constantly unhappy I had no self-control over my thoughts, rather I made the choice to meditate on every negative thought that entered my mind. Upon waking each morning my mind would suggest, *I just cannot keep going, I cannot face another day.* Feeling weak and defeated, my will would choose to agree with this thought pattern and start the day defeated, depressed and overwhelmed - before my feet had even touched the ground!

We all have the ability to decide what thoughts we agree or disagree with, our mind is the forerunner of our actions and our state of mind will determine our daily outcome. Every moment of everyday we are faced with choices. For me my choices, when in depression, would begin first thing in the morning; get out of bed or pull the covers over my head because "life is too hard?"

You may be thinking, "Well, it is not my will to be this way, I certainly do not choose to be depressed, anxious, angry etc." It may not be that your will is to stay this way but you can definitely make it your will to get well. We can choose to take action. With depression it may be that you do not *feel* like reading the Bible or *feel* like taking a walk or *feel* like going to the counselling sessions, this is where you have *free will,* the ability to choose what you do and do not do.

Your free will is more than some invisible force that floats around waiting to see what choices we make on a daily basis. In fact, Dr. Caroline Leaf explains free will as being a genetic structure in your brain:

> "There is a point in your brain called the "free will" and it is a genetic structure, there is genetic code. You can use that free will to accept or reject that incoming information. So if you are controlling your thought life, you don't have to just receive all of this input that is coming in from the outside world, from the media, from external and also from your internal world; we've got a lot of existing toxic memories in our head, everything from birth to death is stored in your brain. So you're going to have information coming from the outside, information from the inside and it all meets at this point of the free will in the brain. You can make a decision at that point to accept or reject that information. If you decide this is not good for me and you actually analyze that thought and say, this is not good for me, this

is not healthy. You can reject that thought and it goes out and becomes heat energy. It actually becomes hot air and it doesn't become part of you. But if you choose to think about it, if you choose to meditate on that, if you choose to ask, answer, discuss, analyze to give meaning, you push it into these memory trees of the mind, into the memory circuits and once they're there, they are there for good. Once they've moved into what the neuro-scientists call the magic trees of the mind, once they're there, they're there for good, you can't get rid of them. Then you've got to rebuild, that's the renewing of the mind. Much more difficult to rebuild than it is to reject" (CCSNG).

How do we achieve the *will* to control our thought-life, the *will* to do what it takes to get well and stay well? I believe the answer is Passion. Yes, passion drives our will to get out and do life and do it well. In the life of a depressed person passion is almost non-existent, or at least it lies dormant waiting for re-ignition, and therefore the mind becomes a "free to do as it pleases," undisciplined and passion-less dark place, a place driven by fear.

In the previous discussion on the mind we established the concept of thoughts as "things" and our God-given ability to renew the mind, though before the renewal of the mind can take place we must first use our free will to accept or reject thoughts. It is most important once the will to get well is established that you consistently take action on thoughts that do not support your *will*. From this point you must harness passion to get well. As mentioned, passion drives our will and without a driver there is no direction. Choose today to get passionate about returning to joy, taking back all that the enemy has stolen from you, declaring out loud "I am a child of God and it is my birthright to be overflowing with peace, joy and happiness!" In Jesus' name, Amen.

Passion creates freedom regardless of circumstance. For example, when I was in depression, my will every morning was to stay in bed and literally curl up to die. However, when I made the choice to get passionate about being well again I began to challenge my "will to stay in bed" and to remain a prisoner to my thoughts. I recall asking myself, *What action would I take if I did not have these thoughts?* My answer, *I would put on my shoes and get out for a run,* was a revelation that hit me like a tonne of bricks! In that moment I realised that regardless of how I was feeling, regardless of my circumstances, there was freedom to be found in the simple act of putting on my running shoes. I determined to challenge my depressed will, dragged myself out of bed, put my joggers on and went for a run. I cried every step of the way. A mix of emotions swung like a pendulum, sad with grief one moment then overwhelmed with joy the next. I remember running out amongst the hills where we live, I made my way down a dirt track toward a herd of brown cows. Before depression I would take a daily run on the same route, the cow paddock was my twenty-minute turnaround point. Often I would stop at the cows and enjoy the simplicity of watching them chewing the grass and just being what they were created to be, no striving, just being. This run was different; it was almost as though I had found a long lost friend, a friend I had been convinced would never return … I had found me! When I reached the cow paddock I stood and watched them for a while and all at once I felt "normal," I even felt a bubble of joy in my spirit, in that moment I cried out to the cows, "I am back!"

It is most important once the will to get well is established that you consistently take action on thoughts that do not support your will.

There's something powerful about rejoicing in the midst of problems, by the simple act of doing what previously (before depression) would make me feel good, something in the atmosphere of my depressed state began to shift. Joy is a powerful weapon. Despite how you may be feeling, start to take steps to partake in things that *used* to make you feel good. I am convinced that our joy makes the devil depressed … now there's a good reason to choose joy!

Once I had decided to make it my passion to get well I continued to take action by choosing to get into life, as I knew it. Gradually, the depression lifted and I began to experience hours, days and eventually weeks of feeling happy. Often times I would be overwhelmed with thoughts of giving up, *Joy will never be mine, it just won't last.* Then the Holy Spirit would bring to mind the story in Luke 17:12 where ten lepers were crying out to Jesus, "Have mercy on us … So when He saw them, He said to them, "Go, show yourselves to the priests." And so it was that as they went, they were cleansed" (Luke 17:12-14, NKJV). Healed as they went!

Belligerent faith must become the very essence of who you are, eager to fight for complete healing and restoration, even when nothing much seems to have changed. Just like the ten lepers, you will be healed as you "go." Go out and engage in life, go to read your Bible, go to a night of worship – go!

In the beginning, getting out and doing life again feels forced, the effort required to smile and engage with people is very much a "fake it to make it" charade. Time after time I was invited to a social gathering and would find a lame excuse not to make it. My children would beckon me to jump in the pool or have a swing and again I would give many excuses why I could not join in the fun. Truthfully, I didn't "feel" like it. However, when I made the decision to "fake it to make it," determined to be well again, I would respond with yes! Yes to a friend's party, yes to playing with my children, yes to going to a prayer group, yes to going to the gym and yes to good nutrition. All of these "yes" moments were the precipice of my journey towards complete healing. Behind every yes there was a large lump of fear in my throat. Most times I felt like crying. I didn't "feel" like playing, socialising, exercising, praying or even eating but I did it, I took control of my free will to opt out and chose to opt in!

Wikipedia defines this approach; *"Fake it till you make it" (also called "act as if") is a common catchphrase that means to imitate confidence so that as the confidence produces success, it will generate real confidence.*

Your free will must be exercised in a direction that rejects all thoughts which do not bring life and happiness.

It can be difficult to go through the routines of life as if you are enjoying them. Despite the fact that initially it feels forced, I encourage you to push back thoughts and emotions that do not align with your will to get well and choose to continue doing what *used* to bring you happiness until the happiness becomes real

Chapter 11

Emotions ... Causing a Commotion

*"Emotions are like a spoiled child, indulge them and they'll
control you" Bob Gass*

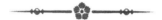

We all have emotions; the key is learning how to manage them
and not allowing them to manage us. Emotions are fickle, my
firsthand advice; do not over indulge your emotions! In particular
with depression, as you first begin to "opt in" to doing life again,
the mood swings can be overwhelming. One moment you will feel
that the depression has lifted and your emotions are high, that is,
you catch yourself laughing or simply smiling and the following
moment you feel completely defeated and easily snap at the slightest
upset. This unstable behaviour would leave me feeling terrible about
myself, it was hard on me as well as everyone around me. Often,
when I would have a good moment or even a good day, my mind
would be consumed with the thought that *this is too good to be true, it
probably will not last.* On the heels of such thinking was an attached
emotion, and a deep wave of depression would overwhelm me
once again. A very valuable lesson I have learned, having suffered
depression, it that it is easy to mistake a bad day/flat feeling as

being a relapse back into a depressed state. Looking back on my rollercoaster of emotions I see clearly now that every moment of my day was based on how I was feeling, as opposed to living by faith. I was being controlled by my emotions. Considering we are body, soul and spirit, if we are to be "led by the spirit" it is most important to make emotional maturity our goal and walk in the spirit as opposed to being led by emotions. Joyce Meyer explains; "We must learn to trust that God knows what He is doing in us. If we feel something in our emotions, that is fine. If we do not feel anything, that is fine too. We must remember that we are in this for the long haul – not just for those times when we feel good, but also for those times when we feel bad or do not feel anything at all ..." (787).

When you have a bad day, which we all do at times, I encourage you to take some quite time with God. Personally, I like to sit and meditate on His promises. In particular, when I am feeling emotionally weak, I remind myself of the Lord's promise; "My grace is sufficient for you, for My strength is made perfect in weakness" (see 2 Corinthians 12:9). Taking time to commune with the Spirit is like changing channels, choosing to switch off a negative program and as you tune into what the Holy Spirit is saying, your emotions will settle.

There are times we all experience periods of being more emotional than usual; however, we are called to operate with the fruit of self-control. If you have a tendency to place too much value on your emotions I encourage you to begin to pray and ask God for emotional maturity. Often I will feel like crying, overwhelmed with sadness and for no good reason! Other times my emotions are full of self-pity, nobody caring about me and the like. Emotions are fickle! There will always be emotional highs and lows, they are here to stay but the key is learning to control ourselves emotionally. We do this by 1) not allowing ourselves to fall under condemnation, 2) resting our minds from trying to figure out what is happening, and 3) taking God at His word, trusting in Him to bring us through it.

Chapter 12

Realistic Expectations

By praying for emotional maturity I am not suggesting we ignore our emotions or that they be buried or suppressed, but we must get them under control. The reality is that suppressed emotions, if not dealt with, will continue to manifest in many ways, sometimes through an imbalance between emotion and reason e.g.; over-reaction, over-sensitivity, anger, anxiety, fear, depression and also physiologically as sickness and disease. Researchers have identified that thought formation and emotional expressions are always tied to a specific flow of chemicals in the body.

Let me conclude this brief chapter with some suggestions for working towards emotional stability. I found these points worked for me and I am certain they will for you also.

Support and connectedness; family and friends, prayer group and counsellor are important for emotional support, I like to say "you need someone to get in the trench with you." Close contact with *supportive* family and friends and/or a professional counsellor creates a safe, accepting and non-judgemental environment where you can express your emotions appropriately.

Prayer and journaling; also effective ways in which to pour out your thoughts. The "pouring out" of thoughts, and the emotions attached to your thoughts, helps to unpack how you are thinking and feeling. In effect, you are "pouring out" on paper or in prayer rather than on the people you love.

Boundaries; necessary for emotional wellbeing. Eliminate one-sided relationships and get serious about saying "no" to anything or anyone that places extra strain on your wellbeing. When you are running on empty emotionally the last thing you need is someone leaching what little energy you have left. I often found when I was completely flat I needed to put in place some firm boundaries … even with loved ones. Something as simple as running a bath, adding a few drops of essential oil and putting up a boundary by closing the door! Boundaries are self-care, not selfish but essential.

Finally, do not place too much emphasis on how you are feeling and keep your expectations real by accepting that you will have some difficult days. In the words of Jesus, "In this godless world you will continue to experience difficulties. But take heart! I've conquered the world" (see John 16:33, MSG). If you allow them, fickle feelings will mislead you and steal your faith. Remember above all else, your emotions do not always convey the truth. When they are causing a commotion you must search your heart, where faith abides, and learn to walk by faith and not by emotions! Take heart, cheer up! Even on your worst day Jesus is still on the Throne and His love has conquered all that comes against you.

PART THREE

HEALING FOR THE BODY

Some years ago I studied a Bachelor of Science. Many of the papers I read were based on the physiological study of the human body however, what caught my interest was the amazing ability the body has to heal and repair itself, a divine design indeed.

In this chapter I will thoroughly discuss healing for the body on a practical level. We will examine what is required for this dynamic creation we call the human body to heal from depression. Physiological needs for healing is a topic which is often overlooked in Christian circles. In my experience with healing from depression I met many well-meaning Christians that were intent on spiritualising every aspect of my condition. Our battle is not against flesh and blood, there is a spiritual realm in which we must contend for healing (see Ephesians 6:12). However, if we are to contend for healing I believe we should not give the enemy so much "air time" that we become paranoid and look for a demon under every rock. Rather, I suggest we must embrace the points discussed in *Healing for the Spirit* and *Healing for the Soul, alongside* applying some practical steps towards healing our physical bodies.

Recently I read a daily devotion penned by L.B Cowman called *Streams In The Desert*. She writes on the issue of confounding physical weariness with spiritual weakness:

> "And what did God do with His tired servant? Gave him something good to eat and put him to sleep. Elijah had done splendid work and had run alongside of the chariot in his excitement, and it had been too much for his physical strength, and the reaction had come on and he was depressed. The physical needed to be cared for. What many people want is to sleep and have the physical ailment attended to. There are grand men and women who get where Elijah was- under a juniper tree! And it comes very soothingly to such to hear the words of the Master: "The journey is too great for thee, and I am going to refresh you" (372).

Along with spiritual laws we also must address the natural laws of "something good to eat and a good sleep," rest and nutrition.

Sometimes the most spiritual thing you can do is rest.

Many biblical heroes, when feeling defeated or simply exhausted, would take time away to rest or seek nourishment for their weary bodies. Jesus would often draw away from people and his disciples to have prayer and quiet time with God (Luke 5:16).

The above devotion is referring to the story of Elijah written in the book of 1 Kings. Here we read the how this great man of God was running away to hide from Jezebel:

"But he himself went a day's journey into the wilderness, and came and sat down under a broom tree. And he prayed that he might die, and said, "It is enough! Now, LORD, take my life, for I *am* no better than my fathers!" (see 1 Kings 19: 3-5, NKJV).

It is clear from the context that Elijah was exhausted - mentally and physically. I believe he had not been eating or resting, that he was running on a spiritual high. He had great victories, revived a widow's son, called down fire from heaven and then found himself running scared from a girl! Sounds like depression. As his body was exhausted, so to his mind became irrational, "Lord take my life" is suicidal thinking! He had already stood against greater odds than one woman and yet he was fearful and perceived the threat irrationally.

How did God respond to Elijah? He cared for his natural needs:

> "Then as he lay and slept under a broom tree, suddenly an angel touched him and said to him, "Arise *and* eat." Then he looked, and there by his head *was* a cake baked on coals, and a jar of water. So he ate and drank, and lay down again. And the angel of the LORD came back the second time, and touched him, and said, "Arise *and* eat, because the journey *is* too great for you." So he arose, and ate and drank; and he went in the strength of that food forty days and forty nights as far as Horeb, the mountain of God" (see 1 Kings 19:5-8, NKJV).

The Lord's care, you'll notice, is always in His wisdom, according to our needs. The primary need that the Lord saw was the need for the body to recover strength: to sleep, to eat and to drink. Elijah had a nature – a human nature, just like our own. Therefore, if exhaustion and lack of nutrition can cause Elijah to have a flat day, then it can happen to us because we have the same nature, a human nature that requires adequate rest and nourishment.

From the example of Elijah it is clear to see the intrinsic connection between the body, soul and spirit. Take heart that the Bible is filled with many great heroes that battled dark thoughts; David, Sampson, Job.!

When our body is depleted, our soul will follow with irrational thoughts, anger, irritability, insomnia, anxiety and depression, which by consequence will make us feel spiritually depleted. The same connection is true in a vice-versa situation, for example, what we allow our thought-life to meditate on will determine our emotional condition and ultimately affect our physical bodies. "When our will reflects His, our emotions receive the best medicine possible. An alignment takes place that gives permission for the body to experience health. A healthy spirit makes for a healthy soul. A healthy soul makes it much more likely that we will enjoy physical health too" (Johnson and Clark, 179).

Often, we fail to recognise a "misalignment" between our body, soul and spirit. As life gets busier we can fall into the trap of neglecting our physical needs as Elijah did and we fall into an emotional demise.

My background in Sports Science and nutrition has served me well in a sense that it has, for the past two decades, been second nature for me to exercise regularly and maintain good nutrition. In depression however, the first alarm bells went off when I recognised I no longer had the *will* to exercise and secondly, I had a very poor appetite and this was completely out of character for the person I am. Needless to say, depression had a firm hold on my life right up until the day (as discussed in an earlier chapter) I decided to put on my running shoes. Many factors led to my healing but the practical needs on a physiological level were of utmost importance to my final outcome. As we go through this section on Healing the Body, I will discuss the complexity of the effects that exercise, nutrition, rest and several other factors have on the human body. It is my hope and prayer that upon completion of these instructional chapters you will be well equipped to step confidently into wholeness in all three areas; Spirit, Soul and Body.

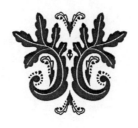

Chapter 13

Depression in a Clinical Sense

According to the World Health Organization (WHO), in terms of prevalent disabilities, depression is the fifth most common and likely to be the second most common by year 2020. The environment we live in, as a Western developed country, is set up for entering into depression. With our fast-paced lifestyles, family breakdowns, information overload, expectations driven by the media, "fake" face booking in social media and living in a culture driven by fear, is it any wonder that depression is on rapid increase?

For a short period of time I was employed as a medical representative. The prescription drugs I promoted were … Yes, you guessed it, anti-depressants and anti-psychotics! Throughout my training with professionals in the field of psychiatry it was often said that depression resulted from a chemical imbalance, but that figure of speech doesn't capture just how complex the disease is. Research suggests that depression doesn't develop within an individual from simply having too much or too little of certain brain chemicals. Rather, depression has many possible causes, including faulty mood regulation by the brain, genetic vulnerability, stressful life events, medications, and medical problems. It's believed that several of these forces interact to bring on depression. The following points are a brief summary of possible causes listed on the *Beyond Blue* website:

*Life events

Research suggests that continuing difficulties – long-term unemployment, living in an abusive or uncaring relationship, long-term isolation or loneliness, prolonged exposure to stress at work – are more likely to cause depression than recent life stresses. However, recent events (such as losing a job) or a combination of events can "trigger" depression in people who are already at risk because of past bad experiences or personal factors.

*Personal factors

- **Family history** – Depression can run in families and some people will be at an increased genetic risk. However, this doesn't mean that a person will automatically experience depression if a parent or close relative has had the illness. Life circumstances and other personal factors are still likely to have an important influence.
- **Personality** – Some people may be more at risk of depression because of their personality, particularly if they have a tendency to worry a lot, have low self-esteem, are perfectionists, are sensitive to personal criticism, or are self-critical and negative.
- **Serious medical illness** – Having a medical illness can trigger depression in two ways. Serious illnesses can bring about depression directly, or can contribute to depression through associated stress and worry, especially if it involves long-term management of the illness and/or chronic pain.
- **Drug and alcohol use** – Drug and alcohol use can both lead to and result from depression. Many people with depression also have drug and alcohol problems. Over 500,000 Australians will experience depression and a substance use disorder at the same time, at some point in their lives (Beyondblue.org.au).

Chapter 14

Pathway to Depression

Irrespective of how depression comes about, understanding the biological pathway of depression may assist an individual to then take measures for the prevention of depression and/or take responsibility for proactively getting well (e.g. good nutrition, quality sleep and regular exercise.) It is not a simple matter of chemical imbalance, rather there are millions, even billions, of chemical reactions that make up the dynamic system that is responsible for your mood, perceptions, and how you experience life. Researchers have developed an in-depth understanding about the biology of depression and whilst there is more knowledge than ever before about how the brain regulates mood, researchers' insight is far from complete.

What follows is an overview of the current understanding of the major biological factors believed to play a role in depression.

Areas of the brain that play a significant role in depression are the amygdala, the thalamus, and the hippocampus (see Figure 1).

Figure 1: Areas of the brain affected by depression

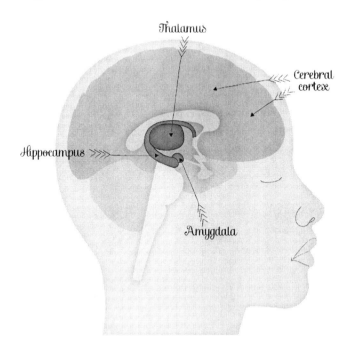

Amygdala: The amygdala is part of the limbic system, a group of structures deep in the brain that are associated with emotions such as anger, pleasure, sorrow, fear and sexual arousal. The amygdala is activated when a person recalls emotionally charged memories, such as a frightening situation. Activity in the amygdala is higher when a person is sad or clinically depressed. This increased activity continues even after recovery from depression.

Thalamus: The thalamus receives most sensory information and relays it to the appropriate part of the cerebral cortex, which directs high-level functions such as speech, behavioural reactions, movement, thinking, and learning. Some research suggests that bipolar disorder may result from problems in the thalamus, which helps link sensory input to pleasant and unpleasant feelings.

Hippocampus: The hippocampus is part of the limbic system and has a central role in processing long-term memory and recollection. Interplay between the hippocampus and the amygdala might account for the adage "once bitten, twice shy." It is this part of the brain that registers fear when you are confronted by a barking, aggressive dog, and the memory of such an experience may make you wary of dogs that you come across later in life. The hippocampus is smaller in some depressed people, and research suggests that ongoing exposure to stress hormones impairs the growth of nerve cells in this part of the brain (Publications).

Increasingly sophisticated forms of brain imaging have led to a better understanding of which brain regions regulate mood. As discussed, beneath the brain lobes lies a region of particular interest, known as the limbic system. The limbic system is the collective name for the structures in the human brain that are involved in emotion, motivation, and emotional association with memory. A part of the limbic system located deep in the brain is the amygdala. The amygdala is the size of an almond; it is this area where we store our emotional memories, especially if they involved stress or anxiety at some level.

When a memory is triggered, whether it be through a dream, thought, a flashback or if you are worrying about something, the amygdala sends a protein messenger, called a neuropeptide (small protein-like molecules (**peptides**) used by **neurons** (nerve cell) to communicate with each other) down to a part of your body called the adrenal gland, which is responsible for the secretion of adrenalin. The adrenal glands are your body's primary "shock absorbers." These two little thumb-sized glands that sit on top of your kidneys secrete adrenalin and also a hormone called cortisol, your stress hormone. This stress hormone goes into muscles and turns into glucose. Glucose is sugar and in this example it is this conversion of cortisol into sugar that gives us the energy to respond to a stressful situation (our fight or flight response). However, if this sugar is not burned up, it turns into a fat that acts like poison and can lead to weight gain, degenerative disease and more. But most importantly, it evaporates from our brain some important neurotransmitters/chemicals that we need for wellbeing and thus, can trigger or intensify altered mood states.

Further, the hippocampus (which surrounds the amygdala) under normal circumstances will regulate the production of cortisol, however an excess of cortisol can impair hippocampus function. No longer able to "regulate" cortisol the hormone can eventually damage or destroy cells leaving a reduction in hippocampus size as cells are eaten away. Psychologist, Dr. Ed Beckham, writes on the possible link between stress and depression:

> "The fight or flight response is a good thing. It has saved many of our forebears from saber tooth tigers and other dangers. But what is good for us in the short run is not necessarily good for us in the long run. And cortisol is one of those things. I believe that our best bet at the current time to understand why stress would lead to depression is cortisol. We do have some evidence that that may be true.
>
> Cortisol like drugs, i.e., steroids, can cause depression as one of their side effects.
>
> People who are given high levels of synthetic glucocorticoids for autoimmune disorders or inflammatory issues have greatly increased risk of going into a depression.
>
> Secondly, we know that long-term exposure to cortisol results in some really nasty effects on the brain, particularly the hippocampus. The hippocampus is the memory centre of the brain. It also does something else. It modulates the

release of cortisol. Long-term exposure of the hippocampus to stress leads to loss of neural branches called dendrites. And it leads to problems with memory loss. If cortisol has a damaging effect on the hippocampus, then it also might have a damaging effect on other parts of the brain.

Current research affirms that damage in and reduction of the hippocampus may lead to depression, therefore we must learn to turn off the stress response. Dr. Beckham puts it this way: "We cannot afford the luxury of stress. If there is anything that we can do which can turn off the stress response, then we need to do it. If we can divert our attention for a few hours, so much the better. If we can fix the situation, so much the better. If we can find more adaptive ways of thinking about the problem, so much the better" (Beckham).

The great news is that you can change how you deal with your response to negative stress. As discussed in the earlier chapters of this book, cognitive therapy, prayer, meditation and journaling are just some of the ways we can reduce the effect of negative stress on the body. In a more practical sense, the following discussion on exercise and nutrition will greatly enhance your ability to deal with stress.

If however, you have been in depression for a significant period of time, the stress of life has worn you down and "literally" worn your brain down, take heart that God in His wisdom has created the brain with an ability to regenerate; He truly does make all things new. Read on to the next section and discover how exercise can promote neural growth (regeneration of the brain cells) and so much more!

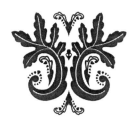

Chapter 15

How Exercise Can Help Develop a Healthy Mind

Despite its proven benefits of improving general health and preventing serious disease, exercise is often a neglected form of treatment for depression. Much research has shown that regular exercise is, in effect, a positive strategy for treatment of some forms of depression. Research suggests that exercise is effective in reducing the symptoms of depression; in fact primary care providers are encouraged to recommend exercise involvement to their depressed patients. Furthermore, "there is evidence to suggest that the addition of cognitive-behavioral therapies, specifically exercise, can improve treatment outcomes for many patients. Exercise is a behavioral intervention that has shown great promise in alleviating symptoms of depression" (Lynette L. Craft). When you consider that up to fifty-nine percent of people stop taking antidepressants within three weeks of the drugs being prescribed, with these statistics in mind, it is evident that exercise may be the only alternative for some (Debbie A Lawlor).

In most cases of mild to moderate depression regular exercise will help relieve the symptoms and potentially alleviate the need for antidepressant medication. Research also suggests that exercise in conjunction with medication can further assist an individual whom has partially responded to an antidepressant. In all cases of depression, mild, moderate or severe, exercise is important to help combat depression and is an essential constituent for the maintenance of good mental health.

Increases and Regulates Important Brain Functions

It is one thing to be told you must exercise, but if you are not a naturally motivated individual the very thought of physical exertion will make you tired. As a motivator, I believe it is important to understand how exercise can help both prevent and alleviate depression.

> "Every day, there is more and more evidence [to suggest this is true,]" says Harvard Medical School psychiatrist John J. Ratey, MD, author of *Spark: The Revolutionary New Science of Exercise and the Brain*. "There are very good placebo control studies comparing antidepressants and exercise, and the effect on mood is the same."

> According to Ratey, depression shuts down the brain's ability to adapt to new situations by limiting the ability of brain chemicals called neurotransmitters (such as dopamine, serotonin and norepinephrine) to foster communication throughout the brain. "Not only is the [depressed] brain locked into a negative loop of self-hate," he writes, "but it also loses the flexibility to work its way out of the hole" (McMillen).

Exercise counters the depressed brain by boosting the production of BDNF (brain-derived neurotrophic factor), a protein that helps neurotransmitters perform their function and also promotes neural growth (neurogenesis). Recent research reveals that individuals with depression actually show lower levels of BDNF in their blood than people without.

So how does BDNF help with depression and how can we get more of it? BDNF can be increased by engaging in regular exercise. Research also suggests intermittent fasting, under guidance, and an enriched cognitive environment also promotes BDNF.

Although the focus here is on exercise, the notion of increasing BDNF requires a little more attention. I believe it is important to understand the significant research behind fasting and increased brain function. Most certainly, consult with a medical professional before you undertake an intermittent fast or calorie restriction. According to a new study carried out at the National Institute on Aging in Baltimore, fasting for one or two days each week may significantly boost brain function. Professor Mark Mattson, lead author of the study and professor of neuroscience at the Johns Hopkins University School of Medicine, has likened fasting to exercising your brain muscles.

Mattson explained that according to research, chemicals involved in the growth of brain cells are significantly boosted when food intake is dramatically reduced.

"Recent findings suggest that some of the beneficial effects of IF [Intermittent Fasting] on both the cardiovascular system and the brain are mediated by brain-derived neurotrophic factor signaling in the brain. Interestingly, cellular and molecular effects of IF and CR on the cardiovascular system and the brain are similar to those of regular physical exercise, suggesting shared mechanisms. A better understanding of the cellular and molecular mechanisms by which IF and CR affect the blood vessels and heart and brain cells will likely lead to novel preventative and therapeutic strategies for extending health span" (Mattson and Wan).

So, how does BDNF help with depression? An increase in BDNF helps to increase neurogenesis (changing of physical matter in our brain, in particular the hippocampus), and this produces antidepressant effects which may help depressed people emerge from their rut. Now that you understand that exercise is the primary key to the maintenance of healthy BDNF levels, it is most important to note that stress is the primary cause of low BDNF! What do we do with stress? EXERCISE it out! Remember, no fasting without the Doctor's approval!

"Feel Good" Chemicals Come Flooding In

You may have heard that exercise increases your "feel good" chemicals? Of particular interest in the treatment of depression is the chemical/neurotransmitter known as serotonin. Serotonin plays an important role in the regulation of learning, mood, sleep, libido, appetite and many other body functions. Research suggests that an imbalance in serotonin levels may influence mood in a way that leads to depression, low self-esteem and/or aggression. Exercise may increase serotonin levels in the brain and also facilitate an increase of other important neurotransmitters; norepinephrine, dopamine and endorphins, all of which exhibit "mood lifting" properties.

Expending energy through regular exercise evidently increases energy and reduces fatigue long term

---

Increased Energy Levels

Next time you feel like taking a nap, perhaps you should go for a walk. In my experience, choosing to exercise when I feel like a nap, has proven to be a better option to combat fatigue and low energy levels.

When you are feeling fatigued, instead of fuelling up on a sports drink, energy bar or a cup of coffee, reach for your joggers, lace them up and get out for some physical activity. I have found that by getting my exercise routine up and running (pardon the pun) led to an increase in energy levels, which in turn gave me the lift required to take action in other areas of my life (preparation of nutritious meals, seeing a counsellor etc.) During physical activity your focus makes a shift away from what is overwhelming you, and the on-going effect of increased energy levels is that it will recharge your enthusiasm for life.

Quality of Sleep

Exercise improves your quality of sleep, with the added benefits of improved mood and decreased stress levels. Regular exercise can strengthen circadian rhythms (physical, mental and behavioural changes that follow a roughly 24-hour cycle,) promote daytime alertness and assist in inducing sleepiness at night. Research is extensive in the area of exercise effectively improving sleep for people with sleep disorders, including insomnia and obstructive sleep apnoea. A National Sleep Foundation poll found that regular exercisers were significantly more likely to report sleeping well on most nights than people who were not physically active. Research has shown that exercise can help to improve not only the quantity of sleep but also the quality: studies show daytime physical activity may stimulate longer periods of slow-wave sleep, the deepest and most restorative stages of sleep (Breus).

Personally, I prefer to exercise first thing in the morning; exercising late in the afternoon or early evening heightens my alertness and I become quite the night owl. Generally getting to bed before 9pm is ideal, as the quality of sleep is greater; my mum has always said, "Every hour before midnight is equal to two hours sleep." I used to think this was just her way of having a quiet house by early evening but there is a science behind it. The *Sleep Health Foundation* concurs with mother's advice:

> "Your best quality of sleep is obtained when your circadian rhythm is at its lowest point (usually between 10 pm – 5 am). Therefore even if you obtain a good amount of sleep (7-9 hours), going to bed late is likely to lead to a large amount of your sleep being highly inefficient. To take advantage of this plan your evening so that you have nothing to do but relax from 9 pm. Then go to bed when you feel the sleep wave: a period where you will feel highly drowsy (for most people this will occur between 9- 10pm)" (van Schie).

In this case, I must admit … Mum really does know best!

A side note for better sleep

While we are on the topic of sleep, I cannot over emphasise the need for good quality and quantity of slumber. Pulling an all-nighter completing work, up with sick kids and so on can bring a feeling of temporary euphoria from running on adrenalin the following day but long-term sleep deprivation is detrimental for the mind and body. On the other hand, balanced circadian rhythms can contribute positively to mental health.

Throughout depression I tried many sleep enhancement techniques: herbal teas, deep breathing and listening to soft worship. All were very helpful but the most effective was "quiet awake time." Where we live we often lose power, and when this happens we have no artificial light, no screens (computer or television) and no loud disruptive noise (with the exception of a toddler tantrum.) In this quiet wakefulness we will read by candlelight or nightlight, play a board game, watch the storm (often why the power is out) and go to bed much earlier than usual. The result in the morning was a deep peace and calm in our home. Somehow the combination of being fully caught up on sleep, as well as the quiet awake time the previous evening, tilted our moods towards happiness.

Because of these experiences, with few exceptions, I make it a rule in our home to have no screens after seven pm. Besides just being a good idea, the quiet awake time has some science behind it. Not only does the light suppress production of the sleep hormone melatonin, but television can actually stimulate the mind rather than relaxing it. I turn off the lights earlier and leave only very few dim lamps on. With everything quiet and the lights turned down, the natural inclination is to go to bed earlier as the dim lighting and minimal stimulation will induce melatonin, causing a healthy drowsiness leading up to bedtime. Melatonin is a naturally occurring hormone controlled by light exposure that helps regulate your sleep-wake cycle and we need lots of it, so to boost production, turn off the screens, keep the light to a minimum and check yourself into the land of sweet slumber at a reasonable hour!

Provides Distraction from Worries and Rumination

While exercise has the potential to transform your body, increase feel good chemicals and keep you feeling confident and healthy, it also does wonders for your mind to be distracted from your worries and negative ruminating. In the very depths of depression I would spend most of my waking hours trying to reason with my unreasonable thinking. Much like a dog chasing his tail, I never caught up with reason. As I mentioned in earlier chapters, my real turning point was when I put on my running shoes and ran out along an old dirt road to visit some brown cows.

Exercise is much more than getting fit;
rather, it's meditation in motion.

I love to run with the sun on my skin, birds chirping, smells of the countryside, focused breathing and on the lookout for the odd brown snake on my path. With all my senses being stimulated it is hard to think about anything else. Often on days when I am feeling flat or just unbearably grumpy with my loved ones, my husband will point to my shoes and "suggest," "You need to go for a run!" From experience, he knows all too well that I am a better wife and mother when I have been out for a run, having left my worries behind and fully engaged in the moment, distracted from whatever had been weighing me down. This works for me, and it will work for you also. After a thirty minute jog, a brisk walk, several laps in the pool or whatever exercise you choose, you'll often find by the end of a session that you've forgotten the negative ponderings whilst being focused only on your body's movements and the surrounding environment.

You may have heard of the term "mindfulness?" It is a form of self-awareness effectively adapted for use in treatment of depression, especially preventing relapse and for assisting with mood regulation. Here's a little tip for you, practice mindfulness while exercising. Concentrate on the feel of the ground under your feet, your breathing while walking, the feel of water on your skin as you swim.

Just observe what is around you as you walk or swim or move. Be conscious of staying IN THE PRESENT. Let your other thoughts go, just look at the sky, the view, the other exercisers; feel the wind, the temperature on your skin; enjoy the moment. As you begin to regularly shed your daily tensions through movement and physical activity, you will also experience an increased sense of control and self-esteem. This focus on a single task, a little "me time," and the resulting energy and optimism, will help you remain calm and clear in your daily life. Whether you choose to train for a marathon or just enjoy walking in the outdoors, get your body moving, take an active role in your recovery, and leave the dogs to do the tail-chasing.

Social Support

If you struggle with the thought of exercise and how to fit it into your life, you may need an exercise buddy. Trust me, you are more likely to get to that gym session if you're committed or accountable to a friend; just be sure to choose a friend that is motivated to move her body and not just her jawline. Besides keeping you motivated, the social support of an exercise friend/s and simple social interaction plays a pivotal role in your recovery from depression.

The Beyond Blue Depression and Anxiety website suggests:

> "Family members and friends play an important role in a person's recovery. They can offer support, understanding and help. People with depression and anxiety often don't feel like socialising, but spending time alone can make a person feel cut off from the world, which makes it harder to recover. That's why it's important for them to take part in activities with family members and close friends, and to accept social invitations, even though it's the last thing they may want to do. Staying connected with people helps

increase levels of wellbeing, confidence and the chance to participate in physical activities" (Beyondblue.org.au).

Feeling tired and being less motivated in general are two very common symptoms of depression. For as long as I recall, exercise has been, a part of my everyday routine so the motivation for me to exercise was already within. I just needed a kick-start. If however, you are not naturally motivated, it can be useful to have some strategies in place until you gradually become more active.

The bottom line is that regular exercise must be a part of your life if you expect to look and feel your best, so you might as well just accept it

---

The most effective strategy you can have is to commit to someone; contact a friend today and get going. Another strategy to keep you motivated is to find something you enjoy, an activity that you will enjoy doing for a minimum of thirty minutes at moderate intensity on most (preferably all) days of the week. Also a very important strategy to get you going is to make a plan. In my days of working as a personal trainer I would tell my clients, "Fail to plan, plan to fail!" We make plans for dinner, plans for catching up with friends and plans for a holiday. If it is important to us we *plan* for it and exercise should be no exception. Make a plan; a specific time of day that you will exercise and what you will do. For example take a thirty-minute brisk walk on Mondays, Wednesdays and Fridays. Start slowly and build up gradually. The bottom line is that regular exercise must be a part of your life if you expect to look and feel your best, so you might as well just accept it … Now commit to a buddy and get on with it!

Medical advice before you start

If you are new to exercise, are pregnant, a smoker, are overweight, have a heart disease or major health problems, it is recommended that you see your doctor for medical advice before commencing vigorous exercise.

Chapter 16

Nutrition for a Healthy Mind

From a Biblical perspective, nutrition was important enough for God to mention it in the first chapter. In the book of Genesis the Lord said, "See, I have given you every herb *that* yields seed which *is* on the face of all the earth, and every tree whose fruit yields seed; to you it shall be for food" (Genesis 1:29, NKJV). Innumerable are the "weight loss and increase your well-being" diets. If you were not already, it is enough to make you depressed! My thoughts on nutrition are very simple; I believe that the ideal diet should be referred to as a "healthy eating plan," a plan that is sustainable for life. Ideally, your healthy eating plan will be predominantly plant-based, anything out of the ground or off a tree should form the basis of your everyday eating and be supplemented by a small quantity of clean, whole, pesticide and hormone-free animal products e.g. milk, cheese, butter, yogurt, eggs, fish, beef, and chicken. If you consume a well–balanced amount of these foods, say … ninety percent of the time, your health will flourish. So how about the other ten percent, what do we do with that? Well, this leaves room for what my kids call "sometimes food," *sometimes* you may feel like an ice cream after a hot morning at the beach, *sometimes* you simply must have dessert when out for a special occasion! The key to maintaining a well-balanced eating plan lies in feeling okay about having "sometimes food" without feeling guilty or tempted to overindulge. If I was to say "this is what you must eat and nothing else" I have then violated your right to choose (and no one likes to have their rights violated), so by allowing ten - percent of whatever you like, you are consequently empowered, given a "choice" to say yes or no to a small treat. There you have it, *Lauralee's Nutrition Pyramid … (unauthorized edition)*. "ninety percent good and tenpercent not so good." That's how I do it, it works for me and it will work for you also.

So, now we have the basic understanding of what is a general healthy eating plan, let's take a look at what we should be eating for the prevention or treatment of depression. In 2010, a research study published in the American Journal of Psychiatry concluded that the modern American or Western diet leads to higher rates of depression anxiety.

> "… a "traditional" dietary pattern characterized by vegetables, fruit, meat, fish, and whole grains was associated with lower odds for major depression or dysthymia and for anxiety disorders. A "Western" diet of processed or fried foods, refined grains, sugary products, and beer was associated with a higher GHQ-12 (depression anxiety) score" (Jacka FN).

It's important to understand that there are a number of nutritional imbalances that can make you prone to depression. Therefore, part of your food plan must include foods that are particularly good for optimal mental health and brain function. Scientific research clearly indicates that the epidemic of depression as a major health issue is linked to the widespread consumption of a "Western diet."

In a December 2012 review study in the Journal of Medicine and Life, titled "Nutrition and depression at the forefront of progress," the authors wrote that:

[Depression] is undeniably linked to nutrition, as suggested by the mounting evidence by research in neuropsychiatry. An adequate intake of good calories, healthy proteins, omega-3 fatty acids and all essential minerals is of utmost importance in maintaining good mental health. In addition, the link between fast food and depression has recently been confirmed (TA Popa).

Unmistakably, diet plays a major role in mental health; a nutritional imbalance in any of the following areas, which are discussed in more detail below, can possibly make you more prone to depression and anxiety. In my experience, supplementing with Omega-3 fats and B Vitamins, also addressing Serotonin deficiency and balancing blood sugar levels, although certainly not limited to being the only dietary factors involved in good mental health, were pivotal for me on my healing journey. What follows are guideposts, if you will, around my personal approach to diet and nutrition with regards to treatment and prevention of depression.

Something's Fishy

Omega-3 fats are called *essential* fats, because unlike some other substances, they can't be manufactured within the human body and therefore it is essential that you take them in through your diet. The richest dietary source of Omega-3 is from oily fish such as salmon, sardines, mackerel, pilchards, herring, trout and fresh tuna. Other excellent vegetarian sources of Omega-3 can be found in flaxseeds, chia seeds and walnuts. Surveys have shown that the more fish the population of a country eats, the lower their incidence of depression. There are two key types of Omega-3 fats, EPA and DHA, and the evidence suggests that it's EPA that seems to be the most potent natural anti-depressant. Research suggests that Omega-3 is related to a number of biological processes that are associated with brain functioning. In particular, these good fats are needed to build the brain's neural connections, as well as the receptor sites for neurotransmitters such as serotonin.

How much should you take?

With regard to recommendations for Omega-3 intake for the prevention and treatment of mood disorders, there are still no definitive guidelines. As mentioned above, much research suggests that EPA is the most effective of the Omega-3 fatty acids in the treatment of depression. Depression websites such as the *Black Dog Institute* concur that a 1gram/day dose is efficacious for a marked improvement in mood. Personally, I take a blend of Omega-3s in capsule form, usually 2 capsules at breakfast (approximately 700mg EPA and 500mg DHA). During an episode of severe depression however, I would recommend 1gram/day of pure or majority EPA. Finally, be sure to choose a good quality product that clearly states the oil has been mercury, dioxin and PCB [Polychlorinated Biphenyl] tested (these are by-products of various industrial processes, and are commonly regarded as highly toxic compounds) and preferably one that is odourless without the use of artificial surfactants.

Safety note

As Omega-3 can have blood-thinning effects at high doses, you should seek medical advice before taking doses of 3 grams or more per day. It is also recommended that you seek medical advice about Omega-3 supplementation if you are taking an anticoagulant medication such as Warfarin (Omega-3 and Mood Disorders).

Beat the Blues with a Boost of "B"

B vitamins are important for nervous system function and the production of energy from food as well as various metabolic processes. Most often B vitamins are considered "anti-stress" nutrients that help to relieve anxiety and treat depression. Of particular interest are Niacin (B3), pyridoxine (B6) and folic acid (B9) all of which work with the amino acid tryptophan to produce serotonin, the "feel-good" chemical we discussed earlier. We also have Vitamin B12 (Cyanocobalamin), which aids in maintaining the myelin that surrounds nerve cells, enhances mental ability and is crucial for the formation of red blood cells.

Like most vitamins, B group vitamins can't be made by the body, instead, they must be consumed from food or supplements. Also, seeing as they are water-soluble, these vitamins cannot be stored by the body and therefore have to be consumed regularly in the diet.

You'll find niacin (B3) in red meat, poultry, pork, fish, eggs, cow's milk, fortified hot and cold cereals, and peanuts. A wide variety of foods contain pyridoxine (B6,) including potatoes, bananas, beans, seeds, nuts, red meat, poultry, fish, eggs, spinach, and fortified cereals. Good sources of folic acid (B9) include green leafy vegetables, legumes, seeds, liver, poultry, eggs, cereals and citrus fruits. As of September 2009, all flour used in bread making (except for flour to be used in breads listed as "organic") has been fortified with folic acid. Vitamin B12 is found naturally in fish, red meat, poultry, milk, cheese, and eggs (almost anything of animal origin), and also added to some breakfast cereals.

Along with food based vitamin B, a good quality supplement may be helpful in providing you with a B boost. Bear in mind however, synthetic vitamins, although beneficial in some cases, lack the natural design of food based vitamins and a vitamin supplement is not intended to replace a well-balanced diet. Despite the proven benefits of vitamin supplementation our bodies require optimum levels of nutrients as they occur naturally in food. In its natural form, such as in plant food, a B vitamin is not only 100 percent safe and non-toxic; it is very unlikely that it will ever be absorbed in excess.

How Much Should You Take?

Recommended daily intake (RDI) by the Australian Government National Health and Medical Research Council (NHMRC) suggest that generally, folate supplementation is recommended at 400μg/day, Niacin is 14mg/day, B6 at 1.3mg/day and B12 at 2.4 μg.

The good news is that vitamin B deficiency levels can be, in many cases, normalised through diet and vitamin supplementation. So it makes sense to both eat wholefoods, fruits, vegetables and nuts and seeds that are high in these nutrients and be supplementing with a good quality multivitamin.

Safety Note

It is important not to self-diagnose a vitamin deficiency because some vitamins can be toxic if taken incorrectly. See your doctor or dietician for advice.

Chapter 17

Serotonin Deficiency

Serotonin is made in the body and brain from an amino acid called tryptophan. It is often thought of as our "happy hormone." Serotonin levels have a pronounced influence over mood, emotions, memory, food cravings (for me it's a bowl of cereal at 3am,) pain tolerance, sleep habits, self-esteem, and body temperature regulation to name a few. For my part, serotonin deficiency is something I cannot afford to risk; therefore I purposefully boost serotonin levels as often as possible through good nutrition, sunlight exposure and regular exercise. Let's take a further look at how you can increase this "happy hormone."

How do we boost Serotonin levels?

We may experience low serotonin levels if our diet is insufficient in protein, have a deficiency of vitamins, through extreme dieting, digestive disorders and also from stress.

Nutrition and Supplementation

Production of serotonin is linked to the availability of vitamin B6 (also known as pyridoxine) and the amino acid tryptophan. Major sources of vitamin B6 include cereal grains, legumes, vegetables (carrots, spinach, peas and potatoes) milk, cheese, eggs, fish, liver, meat and flour. Vitamin B6 is often used with other B vitamins in vitamin B complex formulas; you may want to consider supplementing with a high potency vitamin B complex.

Tryptophan is an essential amino acid; "essential" meaning you need to get it from your diet because your body cannot produce it. Amidst many other important functions, our body uses tryptophan to make serotonin. Fortunately tryptophan is found in many common foods, including meats, seeds, nuts, eggs and dairy. When my appetite was quite diminished during depression I recall feeling as though all I could stomach was eggs, in fact I started to crave eggs! I believe this was my body knowing just what was needed to aid my healing. What is your body saying? Learn to differentiate by what your body needs and what is comfort eating. I recall at times eating refined sweet foods for comfort then feeling guilty for having done so and *then* feeling shame and finishing up feeling more depressed!

Along with eating serotonin-boosting foods, you may want to try mood enhancing supplements. Mood enhancing supplements are to be considered with caution for example St John's Wort. Although it is by far my favoured herb for the treatment of depression, it is very important to note that Extracts of St John's Wort can powerfully interact with the cytochrome P450 enzyme system (the liver's enzyme system; where medications, nutrients and herbal remedies are metabolised) and therefore can affect the way many prescription medicines work, including the oral contraceptive pill. For this reason, it may not be an appropriate choice for many people, particularly those who take other medications.

If you are experiencing mild to moderate depression, I would recommend with caution St. John's Wort or SAMe. Also known as S-adenosylmethionine. This is a synthetic form of a compound formed naturally in the body from the essential amino acid methionine and adenosine triphosphate (ATP), the energy-producing compound found in all cells in the body.

Although I have not personally taken SAMe, I know of others that that have utilised it with sound results. It is believed that SAMe increases the availability of the neurotransmitters serotonin and dopamine, both of which enhance mood. Once again, if you are considering using supplements or alternative medicine always speak with your Doctor FIRST!

Safety Note:

Please be sure to consult your medical physician before taking any mood enhancing supplements. If you are already taking prescription medication, these supplements may alter the effectiveness of prescribed medications and/or cause serious side effects.

Prescription Medication

Anti-depressant drugs, prescribed by a medical professional, are also intended to increase serotonin levels. Your doctor may refer to these as a selective serotonin re-uptake inhibitor (SSRI) or tricyclic antidepressant. In my experience I was able to treat the depression without the use of medication. We will discuss this option further in the Medical Approach part of this chapter.

Exercise and Sunlight

A very effective and natural approach to promote serotonin levels is one which we are mostly all aware of. Yes you guessed it, exercise!

Despite that when serotonin levels are low you may not "feel" like exercise, remind yourself of what's important and get moving. Likewise, sunlight is a quick and easy way to boost your mood. There is a type of depression known as Seasonal Affective Disorder (SAD), which is associated with the seasons from late Autumn and Winter months. SAD is thought to be caused by the lack of exposure to natural light and more likely to be found in countries with shorter days and longer periods of darkness, such as in the cold climate areas. Now there is a great reason for you to head out for an early morning walk, even in the cool weather, to jumpstart your mood for the entire day.

Stress Management

Finally, get to work at reducing your stress levels (but don't stress about it.) High levels of constant worry and anxiety will lead to an increase in the stress hormone, cortisol, which subsequently leaches the body of serotonin. When we assess our current lifestyle against the causal factors of serotonin depletion, is it any wonder many of us suffer from low levels of this very important chemical. So how do we reduce stress? Firstly, you need to let go of worry, which is the primary source of stress. Stress management is one of the foremost steps you can take in the direction of attaining good health for your body, soul and spirit. Bear with me here while I focus our attention away from serotonin levels and onto managing stress levels. God is very clear in the Bible what he thinks about worry. Philippians 4:6 says, "Do not fret *or* have any anxiety about anything ..." (AMP).

Pastor Rick Warren of Saddleback Church hosts an online devotional "Daily Hope" and here's what he has to say on worry:

> **"Worry is unreasonable** for a couple of reasons. First, worry exaggerates the problem. Have you noticed if somebody says something bad about you, the more you think about it, the bigger it gets? Second, worry doesn't work. To worry about something you can't change is useless. And to worry about something you can change is stupid. Just go change it!
>
> **Worry is unnatural.** There are no born worriers. You might think you are, but you're not. Worry is something you learned. Since worry is unnatural, it's also unhealthy. Your body wasn't designed to handle worry. When people say, "I'm worried sick," they're telling the truth. Doctors say a lot of people could leave the hospital today if they knew how to get rid of guilt, resentment, and worry. Proverbs 14:30 says, "A peaceful heart leads to a healthy body" (NLT).
>
> **Worry is unhelpful.** Worry cannot change the past, and worry cannot control the future. All it does is mess up today. The only thing that worry changes is you. It makes you miserable! It's never solved a problem. It's unhelpful.
>
> **Worry is unnecessary.** God made you, he created you, he saved you, and he put his Spirit in you. Don't you think he's going to take care of your needs? There's no need to worry (Warren).

So let's re-cap here, the first step in reducing stress is to refuse to worry about anything. Why? Because worry is unreasonable, unnatural, unhelpful, and unnecessary.

The Bible says in 1 Peter 5:7 that "You can throw the whole weight of your anxieties upon him, for you are his personal concern" (AMP). God personally cares about you and for your needs. You know all those things you're stressing, anxious, and worried about? Let it go. Give it to God.

Chapter 18

Blood Sugar Balance

Have you ever noticed just how grumpy you can get when you're hungry? No sooner does my tummy rumble and without reservation my mood jumps on the irritability swing and oh does it *swing* if it's been awhile since my last morsel of food. One of many reasons for these mood swings is an imbalance in blood sugar levels; there is a direct association between mood and blood sugar balance.

When we ingest carbohydrate foods (e.g. bread, pasta, cakes etc.) they are broken down and converted into glucose; glucose is then absorbed into your bloodstream through the intestinal wall and transported as energy around the body. Above all, the brain requires a steady supply of glucose as its main source of energy and to maintain healthy function. Glucose is the only fuel normally used by brain cells. Since the neurons of the brain cannot store glucose, like the muscles and liver, they depend on the bloodstream to deliver a constant supply of this precious fuel.

However, when we eat erratically, a biscuit here and a pie there, alongside consumption of an excess of refined sugar and carbohydrates (white bread, pasta or other highly processed foods), the supply of glucose suddenly spikes and then later drops relatively low. This peak and trough pattern of glucose supply results in uneven blood sugar levels to the body and brain that has a domino effect on our mood and overall health.

As the blood sugar suddenly drops we will experience an uneven mood, potentially fatigue, irritability, dizziness, insomnia, absent-mindedness, anxiety and depression, to name a few. Since the brain depends on an even supply of glucose it is no surprise to find that sugar has been implicated in aggressive behaviour, anxiety, depression, and fatigue.

Refined foods, sugars and starches (meaning white bread, white rice and most processed foods) are not only stripped of vitamins and minerals but these foods also deplete your body's own store of vitamins. Research suggests that this is one reason regularly consuming refined foods is linked to depression. What happens is that our mood enhancing B vitamins in particular are leached from the body, as the process of converting the sugar they contain into energy, requires B vitamins. *Food For The Brain*, an online not for profit educational charity, cites the British Journal of Psychiatry in relation to processed foods and depression: " … a study of 3,456 middle-aged civil servants, published in British Journal of Psychiatry found that those who had a diet which contained a lot of processed foods had a 58 percent increased risk for depression, whereas those whose diet could be described as containing more whole foods had a 26% reduced risk for depression" (Foodforthebrain.org).

How do we level out blood sugar?

The best way to keep your blood sugar level balanced is to eat what is called a low Glycemic Index (GI) diet and avoid, as often as possible, refined sugar and refined foods, eating instead whole foods, fruits, vegetables, and regular meals. Also worth mentioning is the fact that caffeine and alcohol have a direct effect on your blood sugar and your mood and is best kept to a minimum..

The Glycemic Index, or GI, is a ranking of carbohydrates in foods according to how they affect blood glucose levels. For example, foods with a low GI ranking will raise blood glucose levels more slowly and steadily than foods with a high GI ranking. The higher the GI of a food, the more immediate spike in blood sugar levels elicited. Most often a blood sugar spike will be followed by a plateau or crash of both energy and mood. It simply makes sense to choose whole foods over the refined counterparts.

The Internet has some helpful charts of foods and their corresponding GI rankings, alternatively author Patrick Holford has written *The Low GI Diet Bible*, a book that explains exactly how to adopt a GI style of eating and also provides scientific research on the health benefits of a low GI diet (Holford).

Understanding the link between consumption of sugar, blood sugar levels and depression will help you become more aware of poor dietary habits. It may not stop you from eating a treat here and there, a slice of cake at a party, of course, but the awareness between sugar and mood will help you make better choices in regards to what you eat. This also helps you be aware that when your blood sugar crashes, there's a high chance that so too will your mood. Here's a thought, if you simply must have a slice of cake … Get your walking shoes on soon after and walk it out! Alternatively, warn your family and friends to "take cover because mumma's having cake!" My kids know when my blood sugar is low and my eldest daughter will even get my running shoes out and tell me, "You need to go for a run." You see, even though I know what to do, I still make mistakes and that's okay, just be aware when you do and strive to keep a slow supply of blood glucose trickling through your system.

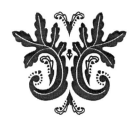

Chapter 19

Medical Approach

Medication to treat depression can play a functional role in the healing process, a useful tool for helping you get back on your feet, but we must take responsibility for playing our role in the journey towards getting well. For example, consider you have a broken leg that has just been taken from the cast, while the cast was in place the bone in your leg was healing, however once the cast is removed you must be proactive, take action with post-cast therapy in order to regain strength and mobility and full use of that leg again. Likewise, taking an anti-depressant will also require some effort from you, exercise, eating well and seeking counselling and other therapies that assist your return to wellness, all of which have been discussed in earlier chapters.

Personally, I felt compelled to take every measure possible in treating the depression without the assistance of an anti-depressant. The depression I experienced was the surface of deep-rooted grief and fear and I therefore determined in my heart to deal with these unresolved issues without the assistance of medication. Certainly I experienced moments where I felt completely defeated and that my only hope was to take anti-depressants to ever feel "normal" again. Whenever I reached this point I would go for a walk, have a cry and make an appointment to see my counsellor. In hindsight

I see it was in these darkest moments that God was doing deeper work in me. I can see now that when I felt most like giving up was when suppressed emotions, hurts and fears were being brought to the surface.

However, I am not dogmatic in regards to medical treatment. In fact, I thoroughly recommend regular appointments with your Doctor so he/she can keep track on your progress and prescribe medication suited to you specifically, (should the need arise). I do believe anti-depressants have their place in the management of depression and anxiety. The point I want to make here is that we must consider, when taking prescription drugs, that they are not a magic pill designed to make the depression vanish.

Chapter 20

Natural Therapies

Herbal Help

And God said, "See, I have given you every herb that yields seed which is on the face of all the earth, and every tree whose fruit yields seed; to you it shall be for food" (Genesis 1:29, NKJV).

From the very first chapter of God's Word we are given insight into what our Creator has provided for us to maintain good health. Herbs have been used for thousands of years and for abundant purposes including medicinal, culinary, perfumes, as bactericides, in cosmetics and many more. In biblical days we read that herbs were grown on mountaintops, hillsides and along the riverside. 1 Kings 21:2 mentions Ahab, King of Samaria, speaking to Naboth and requests to purchase his vineyard so as he can have a garden of herbs! I must concur with Ahab, herbs are indeed fit for a king and a garden full at that.

Science is increasingly recognising the value of herbal medicine and growing deeper in understanding the complex nature of the active chemistry within plants. Of great interest is the fact that many pharmaceuticals have been modelled on, or had ingredients derived from, chemicals found in plants. An example is the heart medication digoxin derived from foxglove (*Digitalis purpurea*).

Herbal medicine utilises plant roots, stems, leaves, flowers or seeds to treat illness, prevent disease and for general good health. In my experience with herbal medicine there are a number of ways in which herbs can be prepared; they can be eaten fresh where their natural taste can be enjoyed alongside their health benefits, or if a more concentrated healing effect is desired, the herbs can be formulated into powders, tablets or liquid tinctures (a concentrated herbal extract which is made from a blend of chopped herbs and alcohol).

For my treatment of anxiety and depression I experimented with all forms of herbal preparations and found the tincture to be more powerful, as the tincture is especially effective in drawing out the essential compounds of plants. In addition, the extract is generally taken under the tongue and therefore more readily absorbed into the bloodstream. Should the tincture prove to be too bitter at first, you can add it to juice or you may wish to follow it with a spoonful of honey, using Mary Poppins' wisdom "a spoonful of sugar makes the medicine go down," in this case choosing honey to make the tincture go down (rather than cane sugar)!

What Herbs to Use

Safety Note: please be sure to consult your medical physician before taking *any* herbal medicines or natural *health* supplements. If you are already taking prescription medication, herbal medicine or natural supplements may alter the effectiveness of prescribed medications and/or cause serious side effects.

Hypericum perforatum (St John's Wort) has been shown beyond reasonable doubt to be effective as a treatment for mild to moderate depression. The flowers and leaves are used to make medicine from the plant, which has been used as a natural health treatment dating back to the ancient Greeks. In fact, the Greek physician Hippocrates, first recorded the medical use of St. John's wort flowers. St. John's wort was given its name because it blooms around June 24th, the birthday of John the Baptist. "Wort" is an old English word for plant. Perhaps that's why I found it so useful in my healing journey … named after John the Baptist, now there must be something in that! Allow me to indulge my creative thoughts here, unlike so many of us, John the Baptist knew his mission in life, he understood his purpose, he certainly didn't follow the crowd but rather the crowds flocked to him. His greatest strength was his belligerent faith and focussed determination to fulfil the call of God on His life. Like John the Baptist, if we can learn to live "on purpose," to embrace the call of God in our lives, we undoubtedly can move forward with confidence fully trusting that the One who called us has an astonishing plan for our lives, a plan in which depression has no place!

Be cautioned, as already mentioned in Chapter 17, extracts of St John's Wort can powerfully interact with the cytochrome P450 enzyme system (the liver's enzyme system; where medications, nutrients and herbal remedies are metabolised) and therefore affect the way many prescription medicines work, including the oral contraceptive pill. For this reason, it may not be an appropriate choice for many people, particularly those who take other medications.

At present, even though depression has gone, I choose to continue with a daily dose of St. John's Wort. I have found this to be effective for me in relieving anxiety from daily stressors, helping keep my mood balanced (particularly with PMS) and I believe that it generally promotes a feeling of wellbeing and mood elevation.

Withania somnifera (Ashwaganda)

This particular herb has been used traditionally for more than 5,000 years in Ayurvedic Medicine and is now validated, by both modern herbal research and many clinical trials, to be effective in the treatment of anxiety, mild depression, panic attacks and specifically helpful for treatment of agoraphobia anxiety (fear of vast open space or crowded places). Recent research has proven Withania to exhibit both anxiolytic (meaning antipanic or antianxiety agent) and antidepressant effects comparable with standard drugs (Bhattacharya SK).

Interestingly the word "ashwaganda" translates to "smell and strength of a horse" and has a double meaning: firstly that the herb itself does have that particular aromatic quality, I would say it has an "I need to go lick my armpit to get rid of the taste" kind of aroma, and secondly, because traditional belief is that consumption can help it's user gain a horse-like strength and vitality. Rest assured, if you take this herb, you will not smell like a horse or have to lick your armpits! Personally, I found this herb very calming, especially for sleeplessness induced by anxiety and stress. At the present time if I am feeling particularly anxious and having trouble sleeping I will switch from St. John's Wort to a Withania complex, this I feel puts a plug on the stress-induced insomnia and assists in generally coping with life's ups and downs.

Aromatherapy

Aromatherapy is the art and science of blending essential oils for therapeutic, cosmetic and mood enhancing applications. Each essential oil has its own unique therapeutic properties, exhibiting highly aromatic extracts taken from tiny oil glands in the flowers, roots, stalks, bark, seeds, leaves, gum or rind of plants. In Biblical times essential oils were used for healing, anointing and as a fragrance for the hair and body; in fact the Hebrew word for anointing means to rub or massage a person with oil. Now this wasn't just a bottle of vegetable oil poured over someone, we know this by the anointing oil recipe the Lord gave to Moses in Exodus 30:22-31, where the Israelites were instructed to make anointing oil with myrrh, fragrant cane, cinnamon and cassia in a medium of olive oil. The Bible mentions aroma and incense throughout the scriptures. Frankincense, my favourite, was added to the grain offering as "a soothing aroma to the Lord" (Leviticus 2:1-2, NKJV). In Matthew 2:11 we read how the wise men brought gifts of Frankincense and Myrrh to the new born Jesus and in the Gospel of John, Mary, sister of Lazarus, took a pint of nard, also called Spikenard, a very costly essential oil, and anointed the feet of Jesus (John 12:3). There are many examples of essential oils being used in Biblical times. Often, I have considered the Garden of Eden filled with aromatic scents from every beautiful flower, plant and tree that our Loving Father created for us, truly a kaleidoscope of colour and aroma and all created with us in mind. In a flower we see beauty for our eyes to behold, oil with healing properties for our bodies, and aroma that can enhance our mood, be it to calm the mind or uplift our spirits. It is not by chance that God created the flowers, plants and trees, some simply to gaze upon their beauty and others with distinctive healing properties; from lavender for an insect bite to arnica for a bruise!

Personally, I have found aromatherapy to be an easy and effective tool for when I need an emotional lift; most nights it is prayer and a drop of Lavender oil on my pillow to induce a deep peaceful sleep. During my journey through depression I had a spritzer (an essential oil blend with a base of water) of lavender, bergamot and rose geranium (all indicated to relieve nervous tension, anxiety, stress and insomnia), which I would use every morning, and some days every hour. Closing my eyes I would spray the beautiful blend across my face, breathing deeply and feeling the almost instant calming effects of the aromas.

---

*Our sense of smell is the only sense that is
hard wired straight to the brain.*

Most days when I am at home I will use a blend of cinnamon and citrus in an oil burner to create a "feels like a home" nurturing environment ... a bit like when cookies are baking in the oven! Ever wonder why an aroma, like home baking, can bring a sense of security and warmth? There is a science behind how our sense of smell is linked so closely to our emotions. Our sense of smell is the only sense that is hard wired straight to the brain. When the nose identifies an aroma it travels up the nasal cavity where millions of olfactory sensors are located. Via the olfactory bulb, the aroma is sent directly to the centre of the brain, to the limbic system, the part of our brain that governs our emotions. When the aroma is processed, neurochemicals are released, causing an emotional or physical response (relaxing, stimulating, sedative etc.) Our brains' interpretation of the aroma will determine the reaction.

Essential oils are also effective when applied topically, whereby the oils are applied to the skin. The body absorbs the essential oil, via the hair follicle, directly into the bloodstream. The active chemicals in essential oils are absorbed, just like the ingredients in common pharmaceuticals such as hormone replacement therapy creams and nicotine patches. Here is a hot tip, lavender oil is an essential addition to any first aid kit. It heals an insect bite in a blink and the fragrance calms the bite victim. In my house it would seem that an insect bite warrants a display of drama worthy of Broadway, seriously you would think their leg had been chopped off! Praise God for lavender.

An understanding of the science behind aromatherapy helps explain how a fragrance or applied oil can have some very profound physiological and psychological effects. It works for me, not as some magic potion or an instant "fix" for a problem, but rather in conjunction with other healing approaches for the spirit, soul and body, as previously discussed.

Precautions

When shopping for essential oils, be sure to seek out top quality oils. Laboratories copy and produce synthetic, cheap reproductions of oils. These inferior products do not contain the "fingerprint" of the plant, namely the trace elements which give the oil its therapeutic qualities. Science cannot fully reproduce the complexity of an essential oil of which only the hand of God is capable of creating. Often you will find a range of oils that are priced cheaply and all at the same cost, this is a sure fire way to tell that these are an inferior, and sometimes toxic, blend of the real thing. Pure essential oils will have their botanical name on the label and each essential oil will be priced according to its availability, locality, yield and extraction method, which is why their prices will vary.

Some *general precautions with regards to essential oil use:

- Essential Oils should not be taken orally unless under the guidance of a health care professional.
- Do not use during pregnancy or when on medication without advice from a health care professional.
- Essential oils should not be applied to the skin undiluted, except where specifically recommended. Always test on a small area of skin first.
- All essential oils should be well sealed, stored out of direct sunlight and away from heat.

- Avoid contact with eyes.
- Some essential oils are highly flammable. Keep all essential oils away from a naked flame (Oilgarden.com.au).

Massage

Massage is definitely one of the most effective and enjoyable forms of self-care and when combined with the use of essential oils within the massage oil, massage treatments serve to bring healing for the spirit, soul and body.

There are various techniques and approaches. Personally, I choose a deep tissue remedial massage for alleviating tension, reducing stress levels and enhancing my sense of wellbeing. A regular, once a month, massage is like taking the car in for a tune up, something you should do to prevent against future breakdowns! For a moment you can switch off from the stress of life as the tension is swept away.

In depression, massage played a key role in my feeling "grounded." My experience of depression was, in particular, a loss of feeling for anything or anyone – a numbing to life. I recall massage treatments literally awakening my senses. Research on the benefits of massage for depression and anxiety concurs that massage therapy has a positive effect on the body's biochemistry. A review of more than a dozen massage studies, conducted by the Touch Research Institute at the University of Miami School of Medicine, supported the efficacy of massage. In the series of studies which included about 500 men, women, and children with depression or stress problems, researchers measured the stress hormone cortisol in participants before and immediately after massage and found that the therapy lowered levels by up to fifty-three percent (cortisol can drive up blood pressure and blood sugar levels and suppress the immune system.) In addition to these positive findings, they also showed that massage increased serotonin and dopamine; neurotransmitters that help reduce depression (www6.miami.edu). Once again I suggest you consult your health professional or Doctor if you have any preexisting health conditions to which a massage treatment may be considered a contraindication.

If you do not already, I implore you to make massage a regular part of your wellbeing regime. Repeat after me, "Self-care is not selfish it is essential." Besides being good for mental health, massage will lengthen your muscles, increase circulation, decrease your blood pressure, relieve headaches and insomnia and the list goes on! I so love massage that I completed a two-year Diploma in Remedial Massage and I must say it was the most rewarding two years of study I have yet done. Oh, and the practical sessions; well, one must receive regular treatments for fellow students to develop their skills ... friends with benefits? Don't mind if I do! Now put a bookmark in this page, go pick up the phone and book yourself in with a PROFESSIONAL, fully qualified massage therapist (do be aware of dodgy "dark lane" or "sensual" practitioners!).

PART FOUR

HEALING FOR THE SPIRIT

Chapter 21

Doubt Your Doubt and Believe Your Belief

Faith and doubt are not opposites; in fact, they're often part of the same journey. When we wrestle with doubts, not just our own, but those of our friends, family and strangers, we eventually come to a position of stronger faith. We find ourselves well able to provide answers to the sceptics and at the same time have a deeper understanding of those who doubt. In his book *The Reason for God*, pastor and author, Timothy Keller suggests we look at doubt in a radical new way. He suggests that we see doubt as normal and perhaps even welcome our doubts as building blocks to a stronger foundation of faith. "A faith without some doubt is like a human body without any antibodies in it. People who blithely go through life too busy or indifferent to ask hard questions about why they believe as they do will find themselves defenseless against either the experience of a tragedy or the probing questions of a smart skeptic" (Keller).

Keller implores believers to look for reasons behind their faith. Failing to do so, he writes, "A person's faith can collapse almost overnight if she has failed over the years to listen patiently to her own doubts, which should only be discarded after long reflection." Personally, my faith has been lukewarm for most of my adult life. Up until I experienced the tragedy of losing my children, faith for me was something I had inherited, a set of beliefs that were passed on by my parents. Amidst great pain and sorrow my faith *did* "collapse overnight." I carried doubt and unbelief for at least two years and believed my doubts were an abomination to God. I was certain God would not heal me from depression so long as I was consumed with doubts about who He was and the promises in His word. Doubt, I considered, was sin … wasn't it? Not according to Jesus. Let me introduce you to my favourite disciple, Thomas, also known as "doubting Thomas." His story resonates with many of us that have battled with reasoning, doubt and unbelief.

In the gospel of John 20:14, Jesus appeared to Mary in the garden. Further along, in verse 19, Jesus goes to the room where the rest of his disciples are huddled together behind locked doors, for fear of the Jewish leaders. And suddenly, Jesus appears despite the locked doors, and he says, "Peace be with you" (John 20:20, NKJV). After he said this, he showed them his hands and side. The disciples were overjoyed when they saw the Lord. And they believed!

Now, Thomas, for whatever reason we do not know, was missing when Jesus first appeared. Notice in the following verses the grace of Jesus, as He was faithful to accommodate Thomas, even in his unbelief.

> "²⁴ Now Thomas (also known as Didymus), one of the Twelve, was not with the disciples when Jesus came. ²⁵ So the other disciples told him, "We have seen the Lord!" but he said to them, "Unless I see the nail marks in his hands and put my finger where the nails were, and put my hand into his side, I will not believe.
>
> ²⁶ A week later his disciples were in the house again, and Thomas was with them. Though the doors were locked,

Jesus came and stood among them and said, "Peace be with you!" [27] Then he said to Thomas, "Put your finger here; see my hands. Reach out your hand and put it into my side. Stop doubting and believe"(John 20:24 -27, NKJV).

In the end it was his doubt, his desire to know Jesus for himself, which brought Thomas to his faith. It is easy to see from this example that faith and doubt are not opposites. It is possible to have faith through doubt or to believe through unbelief. Faith and indifference are more opposite than faith and doubt. Doubt is often a key part of the journey of faith. It's a detour, if you will, along the path of faith. I assure you, when you find yourself taking a "doubt detour," you're certainly not alone! And most importantly, you must know and believe that it's not an indication of you being a bad Christian or an unbeliever. God will bless and honour the very little faith you do have, no matter how weak or how small. I firmly believe that experiencing doubt is a good indication that you are taking your relationship with God seriously enough to be honest, no longer kidding yourself that you are "Holier than thou." You are a real person, searching for real reasons to believe. The acknowledgement and processing of doubts will fortify your faith, settle your reasoning and take you to places in Him that you may not have experienced, had you not searched for a deeper meaning to why you believe in Jesus Christ.

Not being able to fully comprehend God is frustrating. At times I have felt overwhelmed with the thought of never having all the answers. The idea of walking by faith and not by sight is, at times, a struggle for me. Eventually, I bring my thoughts back to the simple truth, there is no way we will ever grasp the concept of God and all He is this side of eternity, and if God could be comprehended by you and me, would that make Him God or perhaps just another historical figure, an outstanding moral teacher? In his book *Crazy Love*, author Francis Chan illustrates the chasm of difference between the smallness of our mind and the inability to comprehend God: " … it is ridiculous for us to think we have the right to limit God to something we are capable of comprehending. What a stunted, insignificant *god* that would be! If my mind is the size of a soda can and God is the size of all the oceans, it would be stupid for me to say He is only the small amount of water I can scoop into my little can. God is so much bigger, so far beyond our time-encased, air/food/sleep-dependent lives" (33).

In all honesty, my faith waivers from day to day. I go from being on fire for the things of God to being quite blasé about my faith. God doesn't want us to be lukewarm; He wants us to continue to stir up, to fan into flame our faith. It is important that you come to Him and tell him about your doubts. Most nights I walk outside and look into the evening sky for a sign that God is "there." When I am apprehensive about faith in God I remind myself of all that He has done for me then I pray something like this: "Dear Jesus, remind me who I am, help me believe it, show me how you love me, overwhelm my doubts. Thank you Lord that when my hope fades your hand reaches out to hold me up."

Chapter 22

The Journey through Doubt and into Faith

Sometimes I let my mind wander and imagine my life without faith in God. On days when I am tired or feeling emotionally flat, my wandering thoughts settle on reasoning what I believe. My focus moves from being fixed on God to being fixed on reasoning. *What if God doesn't really exist?* Sure enough, I dig myself into a hole of doubt and unbelief. Although I write on the love of Jesus and the reality of my faith in the unseen, there are days I approach the word of God with tones of skepticism. Just as the thief hanging beside Jesus challenged Him to "prove" that He was the Son of God by bringing Himself down from the cross, I find myself on occasions approaching my time in prayer with a "so God, prove you are who you say you are" attitude. When I feel times of doubt and unbelief I am reminded of some of the men and women of the Bible who, although they walked and talked with Jesus, were also at times reticent to believe. Jesus healed a man's son: "Immediately the father of the child cried out and said with tears, "Lord, I believe; help my unbelief!" (Mark 9:24, NKJV).

The cry of this father has brought me comfort over the years, as I felt condemned, like I wasn't being healed because of my weak faith. His faith wavered as he conceded "Help my unbelief," yet Jesus healed his son. A few years back, during a period of severe depression, I dragged myself along to a minister of God for prayer and healing from the despair. After I shared my story he confidently concluded: "Well you are not being healed because you are not believing your prayers." I left that prayer line feeling like a stench in the nostrils of God. Oh how I yearned for grace, God's grace, to help my unbelief. Needless to say, the "minister of God" was way off the mark. Like many, he was so caught up in his performance-based religion he failed to hear the heart of God for my situation. Just like the father in this scripture I had a measure of faith, although extremely small, it was still a measure and the God in the Gospels is a God of grace, His grace says to my unbelief, "I will honour whatever faith you have."

I recently read an article in a blog titled *Daily Exegesis*. Here the author builds on the tension between faith and doubt that we see in the Gospel story and reiterates that "the absence of doubt means increased faith and the absence of faith means increased doubt." It is surely then, merely a matter of degrees. It goes on to read: "In some sense, the man's cry reflects all of us, all of our conflict, the cry of our condition - including that of the disciples … The presence of doubt does not imply the absence of faith. Christ honors whatever faith we have and will increase faith when we sincerely desire Him" (Lord, I Believe; Help My Unbelief).

When I am troubled and life is too much, I question: "God why? Where are you in this? Do you even care? Are you really there?" God doesn't retaliate or become angry with my questions. When I turn my back on Him and my faith is pitiful and weak, He draws near to me and whispers quietly … "Do you trust me?" By the time I finish digging myself into a pit of hopelessness and despair, uncertain if I can trust in the One, I begin to think along the lines of Peter. When many walked away from following Jesus, He asked

the Twelve were they going to leave also? Peter responded: " ...
Lord, to whom shall we go? You have the words of eternal life"
(John 6:68, NKJV).

***In order for faith to grow I must be challenged
in areas that require me to have faith.***

Faith is a journey. We don't just receive Jesus into our lives and then
sit around and wait for eternity. In order for faith to grow I must be
challenged in areas that require me to have faith. For me, believing
and trusting in Jesus has been one of those challenges. Daily, I
must take God at His word, yield myself to Him and believe He
has a good plan for my life. An elderly friend of mine takes delight
in reminding me: "He lights the path of our future, rest assured.
Although we have no idea what the future holds we do know who
holds it."

Life's a battle; our flesh and bones are caught in a war zone. However,
in Christ, we are fighting *from* a place of victory *not towards* victory ...
Jesus won the battle when He was crucified on the cross, our role
is to keep reminding the enemy of the defeated foe he really is. I
believe there is no truth more powerful than the truth of what took
place on the cross at Calvary. The word of God says Jesus, "having
disarmed principalities and powers, He made a public spectacle of
them, triumphing over them in it" (Colossians 2:15, NKJV). Author
Bob Gass writes, "Standing on the deck of a US aircraft at the end
of the Pacific war, in an historic moment never to be forgotten,
General MacArthur walked over to Tojo, the Japanese leader, and
publicly stripped him of all his symbols of power. And that's what
Jesus did for you at the cross" (Gass and Gass).

I recently stumbled upon a Latin aphorism, *scientia est potentia,* and it's meaning "knowledge is power" is poignantly true of your power over Satan. Through the death and resurrection of Jesus Christ, Satan was *and still is* defeated. Knowing this truth will empower you to stand strong against all the works of the enemy. The strength I have comes from knowing who I am in Christ and standing firm in the face of adversity. On my weakest of days a profound strength abounds in me, but it wasn't always this way. In the darkness of depression, almost every moment of the day, I would ask myself: "What's the point? What's the point of cleaning the house? What's the point of having interests or a hobby? What's the point in being a mother?" On and on … until finally peace would quiet my mind – this was God. Often I felt like I was adrift in a stormy ocean, barely holding on, desperately searching for a reason to live; yet all the while He was holding on to me, He is my anchor!

Many people ask me how could I still believe in God and have faith in His love for me after all that has happened? But how could I not? If it wasn't for my faith in God I am most certain that I would have ended my life. God is faithful. Life without Him is both purposeless and hopeless. Life with Him brings purpose and hope. Often times I have felt completely discouraged, the chasm between God and the hurt in this world seemingly too great to bear, but may I encourage you when you experience discouragement, and you will, don't give up pursuing God. Faith is a journey, a lifelong process that over time will deepen and strengthen as you read the Word and allow it to penetrate every area of your life.

When I enter into human intellect and attempt to reason what I believe I am comforted by the fact that there is nothing I can do to save myself, for God is the author and perfector of our faith. It is not my purity of heart or unshakeable faith but the work of Jesus Christ on my behalf that saves me. As Ephesians reminds us: "[It is] by grace you have been saved through faith, and that not of yourselves; it is the gift of God, not of works, lest anyone should boast" (2:8-9, NKJV).

He will surely bless those that seek Him, those that wrestle with doubts and uncertainty will find Him. On the subject of doubt and uncertainty, Timothy Keller, in *The Reason for God*, paints a beautiful analogy of trusting in Jesus despite your doubt and uncertainty:

> The faith that changes life and connects to God is best conveyed by the word 'trust'. Imagine you are on a high cliff and you lose your footing and begin to fall. Just beside you as you fall is a branch sticking out of the very edge of the cliff. It is your only hope and it is more than strong enough to support your weight. How can it save you? If your mind is filled with intellectual certainty that the branch can support you, but you don't actually reach out and grab it, you are lost. If your mind is instead filled with doubts and uncertainty that the branch can hold you, but you reach out and grab it anyway you will be saved. Why? It is not the strength of your faith but the object of your faith that actually saves you. Strong faith in a weak branch is fatally inferior to weak faith in a strong branch. This means you don't have to wait for all doubts and fears to go away to take hold of Christ (234).

Chapter 23

Living in the Light of Truth

*God knew what He was doing when He created you. Man's
opinion has no value or authority against
the decisions of God!*

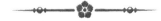

It was during my early school years when the enemy of my soul, the
devil, gained a foothold in my life. With the start of each new day,
dark thoughts of self-loathing would *subtly* occupy my thinking and
by the day's end what had started as subtle, irrational thoughts pre-
occupied my mind to such a degree that rational thought would be
crowded out. From memory, it was at the age of ten years old that
depression set in and plagued me daily. Most school days I would
spend my lunch hour in the library. Depression had taken a firm
grip on my mind. The battles of life are either won or lost in the
mind and the battle for my self–esteem was fast becoming a losing
fight. Relentlessly, the thoughts of insignificance and unworthiness
pounded my mind until they became my truth ... what I believed
to be true about me. I have come to learn that the power our
thoughts have in creating our life experience is far greater than we
can imagine.

Long before the "law of attraction" was a trendy way to *think* and *create* your world, the same "law" was written in the Word of God. The law of attraction is scriptural. "For as a man thinks in his heart, so he is ..." (Proverbs 23:7, NKJV). Scripture has a power and wisdom beyond our intellectual comprehension. In a profound manner, our thinking can impose limitations or chains in our mind simply through meditating on the lies that you have been told, either by others or your own self-belief. If you believe a lie long enough it will manifest as being truth to you, a chain or a core belief in your mind that keeps you from living the life you were created to live. Such chains bind up your thinking. Chains of fear, chains of unworthiness, chains of addiction, chains of guilt and whatever other chain you might choose to think into existence to bind you. It is easy to become comfortable in these chains; accustomed to the limitations they impose. Before long, your reality becomes the thoughts you have been meditating on.

I have heard it said that any part of your life that is not glistening with hope is under the influence of a lie.

Allow me to illustrate what I believe Proverbs 23:7 "looks like." In some countries baby elephants are taken captive and trained to believe they are weak and unable to escape their captor. As a visitor to India you will often observe a chain staked to the ground and then wrapped around the ankle of a full-grown adult elephant. The chain is used to discipline and control the elephant, training her to *believe* she cannot break free. From the birth of the elephant, they periodically chain the elephant to the stake. As an infant elephant, the chain is strong enough to hold the animal in place. It is obvious that as an adult, the elephant is strong enough to pull the stake out of the ground to achieve freedom. Most amazing is the fact that even when the chain is wrapped around her ankle and *not* staked into the ground, she will remain as if she is restrained. How is it so that such a small chain could hold such a large elephant? As an adult elephant, the chain is not strong enough to hold the animal in place; however, because the elephant has grown accustomed to the limitation of the chain, it never tries to escape. Ironically if the adult elephant had knowledge of her power, strength and ability she could crush her captors and everything else around her. Sadly, this beautiful, powerful animal has not been given the wisdom or understanding of her potential. The chain has her believe the lie that she is weak and a captive.

This example is a perfect metaphor of how, much like the chain, and often at a very young age, Satan takes us captive and we remain in bondage to lies and deception about our true worth, our true strength, and our true courage, power and beauty. May I encourage you to take a moment to reflect upon the fears, insecurities or doubts you now carry. I believe many of these have taken root as lies in your childhood and grown to be so familiar to you that you believe this to be "just who I am." The lies you believe about yourself come from the pit of hell. Satan is the "father of lies" (John 8:44, NKJV). It has been my experience that every lie he throws at you, the opposite is true. The only weapon Satan has is fear, it is fear that is at the root of all the lies you are believing. I have heard it said that any part of your life that is not glistening with hope is under the influence of a lie. Fear only has as much power as you choose to give it. Jesus said *all* authority was given unto Him therefore someone has *none*. We give the enemy authority in our lives when we partner with his lies by believing them. Take time right now to uncover the lies and intently search the scriptures for the opposite/ truth. For example a lie might be, "You're going to lose your mind and hurt the kids," the truth however is, "For God has not given us a spirit of fear, but of power and of love and of a *sound mind*" (2 Timothy 1:7, NKJV) [emphasis added].

When journaling the truth you find in the scriptures you MUST also be *speaking* the truth. Make it your own, replace "us" and "we" with "I" and "me." For example two scriptures that I like to meditate on and generally speak out loud, are the following, "*I am* more than a conqueror through Christ who loves *me*" (Romans 8:37), and, "the peace of God which passes understanding guards *my* heart and mind through Christ Jesus" (Philippians 4:7). Let me repeat it again, speak the truth OUT LOUD. Daily confession of the truth, God's Word, will strengthen your spirit and profoundly influence your life as His Word does not return void.

Many women and young girls I meet are captive, depressed and defeated by three common questions that plague their minds as women: Do I matter? Am I valuable? Am I loved? Throughout the Bible the resounding answer is yes! Yes, there is One that says you are much loved and more valuable than humanly possible to imagine. Within the pages of this book you are being equipped with the wisdom and understanding of how the enemy works to keep you in bondage and blinded to the truth of God's love for you. In the introduction, *Content Whatever the Circumstance, w*e touched on how fear and lies only have authority if you partner with them as well as the importance of establishing God's Word, His truth as a rebuttal to the lies. If you take on the wisdom within these pages you will learn how to be empowered by the Holy Spirit. No longer a slave, you will learn the power of the authority you have through Jesus Christ. Defeated no longer you will rise up and take captive all negative thoughts which come to steal your peace and joy. The apostle Paul writes in his second letter to the church of Corinth about the reality of the battle in our minds and how the battle is won by bringing every thought captive to the obedience of Christ:

"For though we walk in the flesh, we do not war according to the flesh. [4] For the weapons of our warfare *are* not carnal but mighty in God for pulling down strongholds, [5] casting down arguments and every high thing that exalts itself against the knowledge of God, bringing every thought into captivity to the obedience of Christ ..."(2 Corinthians 10:3-5, NKJV).

As spiritual beings with a soul, living in a body, we are designed to interact and bond with our maker and with one another. Unlike the animal kingdom, we have been given a uniquely human ability for reason and free will. Using our reasoning, combined with free will, we are very capable of choosing between good and evil. We do this on a daily basis whilst making good moral decisions. With the understanding of your ability to choose you can now also begin to choose thoughts and behaviours that bring life to you; mind, body & spirit. Scripture clearly states that we also have the ability to choose between life and death, blessing and cursing: "I call heaven and earth as witnesses today against you, *that* I have set before you life and death, blessing and cursing; therefore choose life, that both you and your descendants may live ..." (Deuteronomy 30:19, NKJV).

Choose life that you may truly live in the light of truth, the truth of your matchless beauty and worth!

You choose life by choosing to walk out this life journey with Jesus. When you "get it," when you gain a heart revelation of your Heavenly Father's outrageous love for you, it will blow all your paradigms of what you thought love was straight out of the water! He loves you just because He loves you. He's not waiting for you to become any better or for when you become more faithful and holy, Jesus loves you as you are, 100 percent, all the way, all the time and there is nothing you can do that will make Him love you any less ... that's just what He's like, a loving Father like no other.

As I write these words to you, dear reader, I feel His love for you bubble up in my spirit and I know you will feel His presence as the truth of His love for you becomes more than head knowledge but moves to becoming heart knowledge. You are so, so loved by your Heavenly Father and my prayer is that you will believe this truth. Quiet your mind in this moment, wherever you are and whatever you are doing, wait on God and ask Him to show you how much you are loved.

Perhaps, just like I was for thirty years, you are fearful of trusting in His love, fearful that you may get hurt, you may be let down and the promise of being truly unconditionally loved in return is too good to be true. Let me encourage you to ask God to help you trust in Him, just as the father did in the story from the Gospel of Mark. Tell Him about your fears or your unbelief. His love will drive out the fear you've been carrying, the fear that has controlled you for too long now. Know and believe what scripture has to say about love overthrowing fear: "There is no fear in love; but perfect love casts out fear ..." (1 John 4:18, NKJV).

Fear and love are polar opposites. Allow God's love to consume your thoughts and in His miracle-working power, all fears will subside. Think of it like this, if you walk into a dark room then flick a light on, where has the darkness gone? Dark and light cannot co-exist, just as fear and love cannot co-exist. God's love for you will dispel the darkness that has become your constant companion. His love IS perfect love, a love so powerful that it will fight anything that has held you captive. What are the obstacles that have held you back, that stand in your way? God wants to take them and replace them with His love, a love that cannot be earned and cannot be taken away. His love is unlike anything you have ever experienced and once you get it, I mean really "get it," you will be set free to be the beautiful woman He created you to be.

Chapter 24

A Heavenly Perspective

"For I am convinced that neither death nor life,
neither angels nor demons, neither the present nor the future,
nor any powers, neither height nor depth,
nor anything else in all creation, will be able to separate
us from the love of God that is in Christ Jesus our Lord."
Romans 8:38-39, NIV.

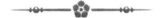

Birthdays come and go. I enjoy the opportunity to go out for dinner with my husband and children but seldom do we make much fuss. A good friend of mine likes to make it a catch up day for all the women in her life, so she decided to invite me, plus another dozen or so women, out to lunch. Normally I would decline. I have never really enjoyed "doing lunch," it just seems unproductive and a waste of my time. However at twelve noon, I decided I'd better make the effort. I walked in half an hour late, tripped up the stair as I entered in my daggy old jeans and a grey shirt ... Hey, at least I was there. My friend rushed over to greet me and then awkwardly introduced me to the table full of glamorous women. I had met a couple of them at past kid's birthday parties but never really connected with any of them. So here I was, perched on the end of the luncheon table with a little voice in my head saying, *What am I doing here? I wonder if they'll notice if I just slip away?* I glanced around at what I perceived were perfect women - hair neat and tidy, pretty clothes, perfect make up, gleaming white teeth behind smiles, all delicately sipping on their fine glass of champagne. Oh how I wished the ground would open wide and swallow me up! Staring at the menu I wondered if people really spent this much money on lunch ... I could feed our Compassion sponsored child for an entire month at the cost of one "gourmet" sandwich! Funnily enough, the menu wasn't going to make conversation with me so I thought I'd better look up and start taking an interest in what was going on around me. During the lunch gathering I engaged in conversation with two lovely ladies, both of who appeared to be "the perfect mum and wife." We all know her. She's that woman in our lives who has everything under control. She's calm, well dressed, always talks so sweetly to her children, her house is immaculate, she carries perfectly prepared home–baked snacks in her perfectly labelled Tupperware containers. Ever been there?

"When we worry about what other people think, we let them control us. We waste a lot of time and energy trying to figure out what other people want us to be and then trying to become like that rather than just being what God made us to be. You're manipulated and controlled by somebody else"- Rick Warren

---

It's easy to get caught in the people pleasing trap, saying yes to everyone's beck and call and even worse, the trap of measuring our own beauty, worth and abilities against how we "perceive" other women to be. Author and Pastor, Rick Warren, says of the people pleasing mentality, "When we worry about what other people think, we let them control us. We waste a lot of time and energy trying to figure out what other people want us to be and then trying to become like that rather than just being what God made us to be. You're manipulated and controlled by somebody else" (*Daily Hope with Rick Warren*). Spending our lives trying to please everybody is exhausting and literally impossible; above all, it leaves you in danger of missing God's best for you. Pre-occupied with people pleasing leaves the mind too busy for thinking about what God would have you do.

Hear me loud and clear ... You cannot please everybody! Not even God can please everybody. I pray for rain to fill the water tanks; my girlfriend has a day off work and prays for sunshine so she can spend the day at the beach. Who is God going to answer? So, you see how debilitating it is to try and be loved and approved of by everybody? The Word of God concurs: "The fear of human opinion disables; trusting in GOD protects you from that" (Proverbs 29:25, MSG).

"Mummy can I see?" My youngest daughter cries out immediately after I have taken a photo of her, then follows with the same response every time, "I am pretty hey?" Of course from my perspective my daughters are the world's most beautiful little girls! My response to her need for affirmation is always, "You are pretty my little girl." Not much changes as we grow to adult women, our heart still cries out, "Am I pretty? Am I beautiful? Am I worthy of love?" True answers to these questions can only be found by looking at you the way God looks at you. When you learn to live in the truth of God's love, not by intellect or emotions but rather by personal revelation, you will grow confident that He delights over you, His beloved daughter. This confidence in His love for you will revolutionise the way you think about yourself. Living in God's extravagant love is not complicated, it is not something you can strive towards but rather simply ask the Lord to show you the depth of His love for you and pray for a heart revelation of what Jesus accomplished on the cross. Your loving Heavenly Father smiles upon a heartfelt prayer, a prayer with words that have been born out of a desire to know and love Him … that's why He created you, to be in relationship with Him, to love and be loved.

In his wonderful book, *He Loves Me,* author Wayne Jacobsen writes on how it is the work of the Father to make Himself known to you.

> "If you came into a room where a two-year old child was playing and wanted to have a relationship with that child, who would have to make that happen? Would it be the child? Of course not! To forge a relationship with that toddler, you would be the one to do it. He'll have to respond, of course, but you would take the initiative. You would find a way to meet him at his level and you would engage him in things that interest him as you draw him into a relationship. The same is true with God. He is further above you than you are above a two-year-old. He will take the initiative at your invitation. Simply ask him to reveal to you how much he loves you, and he will take it from there" (183).

Regularly talk with God, focus on him and begin to recognise His presence. Daily, let your heart be open before him. Not in a religious manner where it becomes a rote chore for you but rather, as you go about your day, ask him to make himself known to you. Spend time reading the Gospels where you will encounter Jesus as a real person, a loving God, and soon you will begin to see yourself, your life and everything else, as He does.

Once you take hold of a heavenly perspective you will stop being concerned with what others think of you, you will get over trying to please everybody and you will be free from the fear of rejection. People-pleasers are controlled by the fear of rejection. Once you decide to dig your heels in and say "no," or defend your beliefs or share your dreams and life goals, you will experience rejection, possibly by the closest of family, friends and even strangers. I have learned, although it hurts, that rejection will not ruin your life *unless you let it.* For most of my life I have been the peacekeeper, not wanting to rock the boat or upset anyone. Now however, I know who I am. I have a heavenly perspective and my confidence comes from who I am in Him, not from what others' think of me.

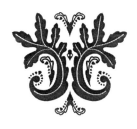

Chapter 25

Past Experiences Shape Your Perspective

Memories of my childhood and into my teen years are much like the "snapshot" taken by a camera. I would often recall the most hurtful memories by viewing them as snapshots in my mind. Replaying what was said and done over and over until I had taken myself right back to those times. What was said to me or about me so many years ago was still interpreted by me as being truth. Eventually, I would have myself in tears, feeling the hurt emotions all over again. Over the past few years I've learned to recall these memories like snapshots on a movie reel, that's all they are. No longer do they hold any value emotionally, they are snapshots of my life and a snapshot does not tell the whole story. For example, if you were to browse my family photo albums you may interpret my life as being fun, complete and pretty well perfect! Let me tell you, your interpretation would be way off the mark as my family photo album is not the whole story and my life has been far from perfect. In the same way, when we replay memories, both good and bad, our mind is left to interpret those experiences. We can interpret from an earthly perspective or a heavenly perspective. One will hold you in bondage to the past and the other will set you free, no longer feeling the pain of hurtful memories. The latter perspective will allow you to view them as snapshots of your life … souvenirs from the journey thus far.

If you've ever tried to "just forget it," "move on" or "let it go," you will know that it is very difficult to switch off from the pain associated with hurtful memories. For many years I tried to wipe away the memories. I sustained a season of being bulimic, I drank too much alcohol, underwent hypnotherapy and experienced loads of new age practitioners calling upon the Universe as if it were some magic genie that would drop into my life whatever I commanded! All attempts I made to be complete and happy were futile until I came to the end of myself, I hit rock bottom, and from there I found myself running back to the arms of Jesus. He created us to be in a relationship with Him and absolutely nothing will complete you until you give in to the One that makes all things new. It was in my quite times with Jesus where I learned about His affection for me, His perspective of me and His interpretation of who I am. A Heavenly perspective changes everything, you are His beloved, He delights in you and longs to see you set free. Just as it is stated in the Gospel of John, " … you shall know the truth, and the truth shall make you free" (John 8:32, NKJV).

In these clear-cut words, Jesus revealed that the key to freedom lies in knowing Him and knowing what His word says about you and your life. Our earthly reference to love cannot be compared to God's love for us. The Gospel of John also defines what love is: "By this we know love, because He laid down His life for us" (1 John 3:16, NKJV). Jesus is saying to you today, you are worth dying for, your worth is priceless and you are loved. Earthly, human love is fickle. People are always falling in and falling out of love but the love of Jesus endures forever. Amazing, awesome … words fail to capture the profound expression of God's love for us. The wonder for me is how would my life change, what sort of person would I be, if I could grasp, I mean *truly believe* the scripture testimony of God's extravagant love for me?

Brennan Manning tells the story of an old Irish priest who, on a walking tour of a rural parish, sees an old peasant kneeling by the side of the road, praying. Impressed, the priest says to the man, "You must be very close to God." The peasant looks up from his prayers, thinks a moment and then smiles, "Yes, he's very fond of me" (Quinn, Yancey and Moon, 22).

My prayer for you is that you will allow God to take your past hurts and be healed of them so that you can really begin to live. In spite of what others say and think about you, may you gain a heavenly perspective of just how amazing and wonderfully loved you are ... And yes, He is very fond of YOU.

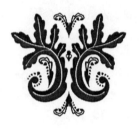

Chapter 26

Conversation with a Loving Father

"Prayer is Conversation with God"
St Clement of Alexandria

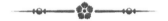

The essence of prayer is conversation with God, walking and talking and taking time to share your heart with Him and taking time to listen as He shares His heart with you. For many of us talking with God has become a pragmatic ritual, no longer a priority but more of a last-minute add on to the all-important schedule we busy ourselves with. Too busy that is, until we come to a place of trial, heartache, pain or sorrow, with nowhere else to go but to the throne of God. In this place we find two choices. We either shout accusations at God for life being so hard. "Save me from this mess," we weep. Or we fall into His loving arms with a contrite heart that whispers, "Father, Your will be done" and trust that He is sovereign over our situation. God brings us to the end of ourselves, destroys our pride, our self-confidence and everything that would keep us from coming to know Him, in order to reveal His Grace. Most of us come to the end of ourselves and wind up on our knees, crying out to God after we have exhausted all options. Time spent in prayer is where God reveals His heart, His amazing love for us. It is in this place that we realise our circumstances do not define God's love for us. Your circumstances may have pushed you towards reading this book, and most importantly, towards a desire to know God more deeply. However, in coming to know Him, through time spent with Him, you will fully understand that God's love is not defined by how good or bad our situation is but rather it is His sacrifice on the Cross that defines His love for you. Your circumstances have brought you thus far and in effect, I write this book to point you towards that love, where you spend time in prayer and surrender all of your strength for all of His Grace. What circumstances have brought you to the end of yourself? To that place where you surrender all and place your trust in Him? In this moment, take some time to contemplate the synchronicities that brought you here, list them down and sit in His presence with a heart of gratitude towards the Father for His relentless pursuit of you.

Time spent in prayer is where God reveals His heart, His amazing love for us. It is in this place that we realise our circumstances do not define God's love for us.

Upon contemplation you will see that what you might consider 'just coincidences' are in fact an unfolding of the blueprint for your life, a plan that a loving Heavenly Father had in place before time began. In the words of Albert Einstein, "Coincidence is God's Way of Remaining Anonymous."

Prayer is powerful, yet so simple and I believe it to be the greatest virtue we have in being a child of God. Often times I have been asked, why pray? If God has a plan in place (His will), then what is the point of praying? My response is always the same; Jesus prayed and prayed often. He habitually rose early in the morning to commune with His Father and in the evening He would often retreat for time alone to pray again, devoted to unceasing communion with His Father. Author, John Macarthur speaks of Jesus' incessant prayer life: "Prayer was the spiritual air that Jesus breathed every day of His life" (16). Jesus' commitment to prayer, His believing it necessary to talk with His Father in Heaven constantly … that is reason enough for me to make it a priority in my life.

Author, Max Lucado, highlights where the Apostle Paul, throughout his letters, more often requested prayer than he did make appeal for money, possessions or comforts. Lucado further illustrates a Prayerful Jesus where throughout the Gospels we see Jesus immersed in prayer:

Awaking early to pray (Mark 1:35)

Dismissing people to pray (Matt. 14:23)

Ascending a mountain to pray (Luke 9:28)

Crafting a model prayer to teach us to pray (Matt. 6:9-13)

Cleansing the temple so others could pray (Matt. 21:12 -13)

Stepping into a garden to pray (Luke 22:39-46)

(Lucado 160).

Our passionate prayers move the heart of God; throughout the Bible we read accounts of the miracle power of prayer. Most certainly, I have been encouraged by the story of Hannah, mother of Samuel. Barren and overwhelmed with grief for her longing to have a child,

> "… She *was* in bitterness of soul, and prayed to the LORD and wept in anguish." She cried out in prayer, " … she

made a vow and said, 'O LORD of hosts, if You will indeed look on the affliction of Your maidservant and remember me, and not forget Your maidservant, but will give Your maidservant a male child, then I will give him to the LORD all the days of his life, and no razor shall come upon his head'" (1 Samuel 1:10-11, NKJV).

Hannah cried out to the Lord with emotion and honesty and the Lord answered. "So it came to pass in the process of time that Hannah conceived and bore a son, and called his name Samuel, saying: "Because I have asked for him from the LORD" (1 Samuel 1:20, NKJV). Unlike Hannah's experience not all prayers are answered with the answer we desire, but they are however, *all* answered by a Sovereign God that knows what's best for His children. We will discuss prayer and God's will a little further in this chapter.

Praying, walking and talking with Jesus would solidify my faith and belief in the power of prayer ... wouldn't it? I feel, shall we say, "normal" when I read the scriptures of the heroes of the Bible. These men and women that walked with Jesus and witnessed many miracles also struggled with prayer. In the book of Acts we read about the apostle Peter, imprisoned: " ... but constant prayer was offered to God for him by the church" (Acts 12:5, NKJV). If you struggle to believe that God would ever hear, let alone answer your prayer, well, you're in good company. The early followers of Christ wrestled with doubting the power of their prayers.

As the church earnestly prayed for his release:

> "Now behold, an angel of the Lord stood by *him*, and a light shone in the prison; and he struck Peter on the side and raised him up, saying, "Arise quickly!" And his chains fell off *his* hands. Then the angel said to him, "Gird yourself and tie on your sandals"; and so he did. And he said to him,

"Put on your garment and follow me." So he went out and followed him, and did not know that what was done by the angel was real, but thought he was seeing a vision. When they were past the first and the second guard posts, they came to the iron gate that leads to the city, which opened to them of its own accord; and they went out and went down one street, and immediately the angel departed from him. And when Peter had come to himself, he said, "Now I know for certain that the Lord has sent His angel, and has delivered me from the hand of Herod and *from* all the expectation of the Jewish people."

So, when he had considered *this,* he came to the house of Mary, the mother of John whose surname was Mark, where many were gathered together praying. And as Peter knocked at the door of the gate, a girl named Rhoda came to answer. [14] When she recognized Peter's voice, because of *her* gladness she did not open the gate, but ran in and announced that Peter stood before the gate. [15] But they said to her, "You are beside yourself!" Yet she kept insisting that it was so. So they said, "It is his angel."

Now Peter continued knocking; and when they opened *the door* and saw him, they were astonished" (Acts 12: 7–16, NKJV).

In his book, *Out Live Your Life*, Max Lucado comments on this passage of scripture: "I confess a sense of relief at that reading. Even the early followers struggled to believe that God would hear them. Even when the answer knocked at the door, they hesitated" (158).

Most of us at some point in our lives find difficulty in believing our prayers, or more so, even just making time for prayer. Life is busy; we hurry through our prayers (when we remember to pray), our minds drift to thoughts of what's for dinner and our focus is scattered and everywhere, everywhere but on God.

God has uniquely created each one of us to interact with Him as individuals and your prayer style should be consistent with the way He designed you.

Prayer is simply conversation with God. There needs to be no set time or location and in comparison to the other tasks we face daily, there is minimal effort required. Yet so many believers struggle with taking time to talk with God. Lucado expressed our struggle with prayer as: " ... you'd think we were wrestling a greased pig" (159). Prayer is an effective and powerful tool and the enemy knows this, he pulls all stocks in an effort to hinder your commitment to prayer. Our adversary knows what happens when we pray, "We use our powerful God-tools for smashing warped philosophies, tearing down barriers erected against the truth of God, fitting every loose thought and emotion and impulse into the structure of life shaped by Christ" *2 Corinthians 10:4, MSG.* Lucado writes, " ... Satan seeks to interrupt our prayers. Our battle with prayer is not entirely our fault. The devil knows the stories; he witnessed the angel in Peter's cell ..." Be encouraged to pick up your "God-tools" and watch as the enemy cowers. Lucado continues:

> "Satan is not troubled when Max writes books or prepares sermons, but his knobbly knees tremble when Max prays. Satan does not stutter or stumble when you walk through church doors or attend committee meetings. Demons aren't flustered when you read this book. But the walls of hell shake when one person with an honest heart and faithful confession says, "Oh, God how great thou art." Satan keeps you and me from prayer. He tries to position himself

between us and God. But he scampers like a spooked dog when we move forward" (159).

So now that we understand the power of prayer, I believe it is important that we adopt the right attitude in prayer. Let me start by clarifying, there are prayer principles that apply to all of us; by reading the Lord's prayer (Matthew 6:9-13) we are able to establish the fundamentals of prayer. John Macarthur points out, "Prayer begins and ends not with the needs of man but with the glory God (John 14:13). It should be concerned primarily with who God is, what He wants, and how He can be glorified" (53-54). When Jesus said, "Pray, then, in this way." He was not saying pray these exact words and parrot them off like mindless clones, after all, He had previously warned the disciples of the dangers of "meaningless repetition." His intention was to give some principles of prayer, a divine pattern to follow, a prayer so simple in form and yet one in which we notice that every phrase and petition focuses on God. This is not to say we shouldn't recite the Lord's Prayer. Macarthur writes: "Memorising it (the Lord's Prayer) is actually helpful so we can meditate on its truths as we formulate our own thoughts. The prayer is mainly a model we can use to give direction to our own praise, adoration, and petitions. It is not a substitute for our own prayers but a guide for them" (56).

Be yourself. Approach Him with your own personality, your strengths, weaknesses and everything that is you. In the book of 1 Samuel mentioned above, we read the story of Hannah, heartbroken and grief stricken, as she was childless in a society that considered not having a child the ultimate failure. When Hannah cried out to God I imagine she wasn't on her knees with head bowed and whispering her petitions, rather the Word says she was "in bitterness of soul and wept in anguish" (1 Samuel 1:12, NKJV). God wants to meet with you; He wants to take you just as you are.

I recall a time of desperate prayer on my knees in the pouring rain. As I "wept in anguish," God answered and my journey of healing began in that one desperate moment. God loves that we come to Him with our emotions, our hurt, our true self; just as a parent does with his child. I want my children to feel they can come to me with all manner of problems, not hide their emotions under a veil of fear.

When my daughters come to me and show dependence on me in my role as a loving parent, I feel fulfilled, my heart bubbles with love that they trust me with their deepest hurts. In similar ways, the parent-child relationship defines the attitude we ought to have in prayer. This attitude is one that focuses on God and expresses absolute dependence on Him as Father, the One who gave us life and who loves, cares for, provides for, and protects us.

Sometimes at night I hear my little girl praying, not some mechanical script, but words that flow from a heart of thanksgiving and faith in a Heavenly Father that "makes everything okay, because He loves me." God is not manipulated by long-winded, rehearsed babbling but rather, He is moved by our heart attitude, an attitude that seeks His presence … not His presents.

Jacobsen recounts, His crucifixion was imminent, "He stood on the threshold of the greatest act of love and trust our world would ever behold, but in doing so he would be consumed" (175.) Jesus enquired of his disciples how they thought he should pray in his final hours. "What shall I say? 'Father, save me from this hour'" Facing certain death, Jesus' attitude in prayer was "Father, glorify your name" (John 12:27, NKJV).

> "In this brief exchange you learn everything you will need to know about prayer and what it means to follow God in this life. For in every situation you'll ever encounter, you will be offered two options in prayer: "Father, save

me," or "Father, glorify your name!" One will lead you to frustration and disillusionment, the other to the greatest wonders in God's heart" (Jacobsen, 176).

In recent years I have recognised that most of my prayer life was spent approaching God with a selfish "I know what's best" attitude. Even worse, I was taught to treat my Heavenly Father like a genie in a bottle who had nothing better to do than meet my selfish requests. How did we miss the beauty and simplicity of prayer? Jesus never prayed in a manipulative, self-centred manner and He never intended prayer to be the way we manoeuvre God to do what we think is best. Jacobsen notes, "If you look carefully at Jesus' simple statements about prayer, you will see that they are set in the midst of our participating in what God is doing" (177).

God already knows what you need, He has a divine purpose for every situation you face, so instead of crying out "save me" or "bless me," may I encourage you to move beyond fear-based praying, disarm your self-interests and enter into a prayer life based on love, for His love will never fail you. Love-based prayers assert trust in a Heavenly Father that is Sovereign and always has your best interest at the centre of His heart. Further, you must put aside all intellectual knowledge about how to pray. Simply take the principles of prayer to Him and ask: "Lord, teach me to pray and to glorify your name in every breath and every step that I take." As you do this He will faithfully lead you in a prayer style that is a natural expression of who you are. Most importantly, stay in communion with your Father in Heaven. Cherish your unity together as you go throughout the day. Talk with Him, take every aspect of your life to Him in prayer and trust Him as He is working "all things together for good."

Chapter 27

Praise and Worship

"Worship is a human response to a divine revelation"
Chuck Swindoll

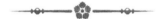

Although frequently used to mean the same thing, praise and worship are two different concepts. I write about the difference between the two because there are times in life when it seems God is absent, or simply does not care and it is easy to enter into the temptation of being angry and bitter towards God. Many times throughout life you will feel there is nothing praiseworthy about a situation, I want to remind you however that there is always reason to worship Him as your Holy, loving Heavenly Father in spite of your circumstances. The crucial difference I want to make is that God is unchanging – this is "who" He is and is reason enough to worship, despite what is happening in your life. When you understand the difference between worship and praise your faith will no longer be a rollercoaster ride subject to your circumstances. Many Christians praise God for what He has done and then when things are not going so well get bitter and angry at God, hurling accusations at Him for "sitting on His hands." I know only too well how important it is when there seems no reason whatsoever to praise God that we must press on and choose to worship Him. Meditating on the unchanging attributes of God will keep you anchored when life's storms cross your path. In the midst of pain and sorrow, may I encourage you to choose an attitude of worship, knowing that God is loving, faithful and always in control of what is happening.

For years I believed worship was what took place in a Holy temple or in church on a Sunday and it would seem that many others still believe there's a special time and place to worship. Worship is more than music; it's a way of life. We worship God by approaching everything we do, think and say in a way that will bring Him glory. It is a lifestyle that's lived according to His Word. Worship is a vast concept, so vast that I find it impossible to define exactly all that worship is. Author of *The Air I Breathe*, Louie Giglio, defines worship as primarily our "response" to God. He writes: "Worship is our response, both personal and corporate, to God for who He is, and what He has done; expressed in and by the things we say and the way we live" (78). So whether it's changing a dirty nappy, working on a mission field or pulling teeth; when you do everything you do to the glory of God, as though you were doing it for Him – this is a life of worship; it is a response to God.

Let's consider again the quote of Wayne Jacobsen written in the earlier section, *A Heavenly Perspective:*

> "If you came into a room where a two-year old child was playing and wanted to have a relationship with that child, who would have to make that happen? Would it be the child? Of course not! To forge a relationship with that toddler, you would be the one to do it. He'll have to respond, of course, but you would take the initiative. You would find a way to meet him at his level and you would engage him in things

that interest him as you draw him into a relationship. The same is true with God" (183).

So we see here, the child responds to the adult who has initiated a relationship. If worship is a "response" then doesn't that, in effect, tell us that God, like the adult in this example, has first taken the initiative to forge a relationship? Because God has first extended to us His grace and love, worship then is how we respond to Him for all He is; as a loving, Holy and righteous God.

In depression it's hard to *do* anything, let alone have an attitude of worship about it. I encourage you to play some worship music, even on days when you don't *feel* like listening to Christian music. On my darkest days, bombarded with suicidal thoughts, I determined to immerse myself in worship music. My mind would argue: "Well, I am too depressed for music, I am not in the mood," but in contrast to my feelings I was spiritually hungry, after all, we are created to worship our Heavenly Father.

Despite how you may be feeling, I want to encourage you to push back thoughts of self-pity, ignore your emotions and feed your spirit. The very second you turn some Christian worship music on, your spirit will grasp it. At first, you may feel not much is changing, but God is doing powerful work behind the scenes. In a profound way the atmosphere will shift whenever worship music is present, as it ministers truth to your spirit the fog in your mind, the negative emotions and depressive mood, will lift also. Worship takes the focus off you and your circumstances and places it onto God, where it belongs.

While worship and praise go hand in hand, understand that they are also distinctly different. In particular, the Psalms show us that worship is based on *who God is*, while praise is based on *what He does*. In Psalm 99:5, David writes: "Exalt the LORD our God, And worship at His footstool— He *is* holy" (NKJV). Worship, David implies, is grounded in "who God is." Praise is often mentioned in the Psalms as a heart cry because of what He has done. Psalm 139 is undoubtedly one of my favourites, it is a Psalm that gives me reason to praise God (when there doesn't seem to be a lot to praise Him for.) In particular, verse 14, where David declares, "I will praise You, for I am fearfully *and* wonderfully made; Marvelous are Your works, And *that* my soul knows very well." Notice the praise is centered here on what God "has done."

May I encourage you, when you encounter times in your life where it appears not much is praiseworthy, turn your heart to God and choose to worship Him for who He is. Worship him as a response to the One who first loved you.

Throughout the Psalms, David often voiced his disappointment for injustice done toward him. When he was being oppressed and persecuted, David cried out, "Hear my prayer, O LORD, Give ear to my supplications! In Your faithfulness answer me, *And* in Your righteousness" (Psalm 143:1, NKJV). David reminds himself of who God is and follows on by what He has done, "I remember the days of old; I meditate on all Your works; I muse on the work of Your hands" (Psalm 143:5, NKJV). Despite your circumstances, God is still on the throne, He is Sovereign, eternal and unchanging, He reigns over your situation. This truth alone is worthy of Worship. As you choose to worship God for who He is, praise will follow and usher you into His rest as a child in the arms of a loving Father. Finally, the lyrics of *Love Came Down* by Brian Johnson, sum up perfectly what it is to worship God when you cannot find reason for praise:

> If my heart is overwhelmed and I cannot hear Your voice

> I'll hold on to what is true though I cannot see

If the storms of life they come and the road ahead gets steep

I will lift these hands in faith

I will believe

I remind myself of all that You've done

And the life I have because of Your Son …

(Love Came Down, Brian Johnson).

Chapter 28

I Forgive Him ... I Forgive Him Not

"Forgiveness is the fragrance the violet sheds
on the heel that has crushed it."
Mark Twain

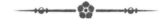

Forgiveness ... If undeserved or unearned you might say, "Well, no one understands what they did to me, what was said about me." From the Gospels' accounts, Jesus had every reason to be bitter, angry and unforgiving. Amidst brutal circumstances He said, "Forgive them ..." Betrayed, falsely accused, whipped, beaten and spat on, he was then nailed to a cross by *them*. As the crowd continued to taunt and curse Him and with His life slowly fading away, He did not seek justice or vengeance. Forgiveness, or as I like to call it, "absorbing the debt," is your first step out of pain. This step involves refusing to make *them* pay for what they did and it is, I believe, the hardest and most courageous step towards healing and complete peace. On the subject of forgiveness, Timothy Keller explains how wanting to make the perpetrators suffer for what they have done will not give you peace. "Cycles of reaction and retaliation can go on for years. Evil has been done to you – yes. But when you try to get payment through revenge the evil does not disappear. Instead it spreads, and it spreads most tragically of all into you and your own character"(188).

It was only a few months ago when I sat in prayer and asked God, "Why am I not completely peaceful and why have you not given me joy like you promise in your word? I am not moving from this chair until you heal me … completely!" I waited for an answer and started to reflect on all the steps I had taken towards getting well; countless counselling sessions, prayer, exercise and the like. As my mind wandered (still waiting for God to answer) I recalled the most hurtful moments of my past and thanked God for healing me from the emotional pain. Upon examining my feelings I realised the memories still affected me, not in a hurtful, saddening manner as they had for so many years. What rose up in my spirit though were anger, bitterness and unforgiveness. Needless to say, God had answered my demanding prayer by showing me that my final healing was to be found in letting go of the unforgiveness that I relentlessly held so tightly. Holding onto unforgiveness seemed to be my last chance at vengeance and justice to those that had wronged me. They didn't deserve my forgiveness!

The issue isn't whether the person who hurt you deserves to be forgiven; the truth of the matter is that forgiveness is a gift you give yourself.

The crazy thing about a "payback" mindset is that the paying back seldom affects those who have wronged you. The unforgiving heart doesn't heal; in fact bitterness and anger controlled me more and more as the years went by. Ask yourself, how does *your* holding onto un-forgiveness work to hurt the other person? Does it really make you feel peace, joy or a sense of true happiness? The issue isn't whether the person who hurt you deserves to be forgiven; the truth of the matter is that forgiveness is a gift you give yourself. In my experience, the hurting one is the unforgiving soul. Much like a snake bite, if you were to be bitten (hurt by someone) the snake takes off into the bush and you're left with the venom (unforgiveness). Do you get the picture? The snake isn't concerned about how much venom you have pumping through your veins; he has gone about his life as if not much has changed. On the other hand, if the anti-venom (forgiveness) is not administered to the victim of a snake bite, her health will deteriorate rapidly and possibly become fatal My friend Nicholas who runs a reconciliation company called "Heart Hacks" explains, "forgiveness is clearing out the record of wrongs from the mess of another person(s) or event(s) that left you feeling, and maybe believing, you are not valuable. The records of wrongs are so vitally important to remove out of our hearts. These recorded moments are authorizing unhealthy patterns and lies to live and have temporary victories in our lives. They rob us blind and right in the open. Removing the record of wrongs instantly starts the flow of unconditional love in our hearts that can never be stopped. It can however be temporarily blocked".

"These recorded moments are authorizing unhealthy patterns and lies to live and have temporarily victories in our lives" – Nicholas Howard

---

In fact, medical research increasingly points to the direct correlation between our thought life and the illnesses that plague our bodies. Science suggests eighty-seven to ninety-five percent of current mental, physical and emotional illnesses come from our thought life. With this knowledge, forgiveness is no longer just "the right thing to do," more importantly it would seem that there are intellectual and medical reasons to forgive. If we do not have a change of mind we can actually make ourselves sick! Long before we had medical proof, the complex interplay between the mind and body was well understood in Biblical times. In a display of wisdom and godly common sense, King Solomon writes, "A sound mind makes for a robust body, but runaway emotions corrode the bones" (Proverbs 14:30, MSG). The amplified version declares; "A calm *and* undisturbed mind *and* heart are the life *and* health of the body, but envy, jealousy, *and* wrath are like rottenness of the bones."

Toxic thoughts and experiences such as un-forgiveness are "rottenness to the bones." Negative thoughts cause brain cells to shrivel and die and this results in a heavy, dark memory. Brain imaging illustrates that these memories are literally a dark shadow looking like an abscess or cancer. Dr. Caroline Leaf, author of *Who Switched off My Brain*, has devoted her adult life to the study of thoughts and their effect on our brain. Dr. Leaf pens her research with regards to close study of brain imaging. You can see examples of these images at www.drleaf.com. The imaging reveals our thoughts and memories as dark shadows, shadows which look similar to trees, some with lush branches and some with thorn-like branches. Toxic thoughts, for example, hanging onto anything that is negative; anger, irritation, frustration, bitterness, will bring about a physical change in your brain, literally changing the structure of your "trees."

Therefore, by choosing unforgiveness, you are building an ugly, mangled thornbush-like structure in the brain. Positive thoughts or love-based thinking on the other hand build thoughts or memories that present as lush, healthy trees.

Simply put, positive thoughts and experiences will induce brain cells to expand while negative thoughts and experiences will cause brain cells to shrivel and die. Dr. Leaf, suggests toxic thoughts build toxic memories and thus toxic bodies:

"Because we are spirit, soul, body and it's our soul area, which is literally the brain insulating the will and emotions that is processing and building all these thoughts into real things, so structural changes are happening in the brain. And whatever is going on in the soul will affect the spirit and will affect the body … if our mind is filled with chaos, chaos will reign in our bodies" (It's Supernatural).

I trust this illustration has invoked you to make a decision to forgive those who have wronged you. Forgiveness will bring healing to your body and your broken heart, do your part and truly forgive them and God will do His part to help you heal from the emotional pain that has held you captive to the past. Like me, you may forgive a person but still have ill feeling towards him or her. The truth is, you cannot truly forgive without the Holy Spirit's help. No amount of self-determination or strong will can achieve complete love and forgiveness. Our human nature is to be led by our feelings. As some of my well-meaning friends retort, "Be strong, don't let him get away with that … it's a dog eat dog world" at the mere mention of forgiveness! I readily admit that forgiveness is unfair. However, if we do not forgive we will become resentful. The word *resentment* literally means, "to feel again." As Philip Yancey succinctly put it: " … resentment clings to the past, relives it over and over, picks each fresh scab so that the wound never heals" (*What's So Amazing About Grace*, 97).

"Forgiveness must be granted before it can be felt, but it does come eventually. It leads to a new peace, a resurrection". – Timothy Keller

---

Despite what the world says, a strong courageous woman is a forgiving woman. Granting forgiveness doesn't *feel* natural, but if we do not transcend nature, we remain in bondage to the past, held captive to the people we cannot forgive. Author and Pastor, Timothy Keller refers to the act of forgiveness as feeling like a death initially, but it is a death that leads to resurrection. "Forgiveness must be granted before it can be felt, but it does come eventually. It leads to a new peace, a resurrection" (*The Reason for God, 189*). Although a most unnatural act, forgiveness offers a way out and as you choose to forgive, I assure you, faith will carry you beyond your feelings and by His spirit, God will give you the courage and strength to forgive your enemies, wish them well and let them go their way. Release your grip on them and you consequently will be set free to soar high above the circumstances which have held you back for so long now.

How do you know if you've truly forgiven someone? To truly forgive someone is to extend mercy, although undeserved, and pray for their happiness. We see this principle in the Bible "Bless those who curse you, and pray for those who spitefully use you …"(Luke 6:28, NKJV). Here's how we know we have forgiven, when we can speak well of our enemies and truly pray God's blessing's upon them.

Philip Yancey referred to forgiveness as being "An Unnatural Act" when he wrote:

> I never find forgiveness easy, and rarely do I find it completely satisfying. Nagging injustices remain, and the wounds still cause pain. I have to approach God again and again, yielding to him the residue of what I thought I had committed to him long ago. I do so because the Gospels make clear the connection: God forgives my debts as I forgive my debtors. The reverse is also true: Only by living in the stream of God's grace will I find the strength to respond with grace toward others (93).

Like Yancey, all too often I drift back into a payback mentality. I must get even! But then I am reminded that as God is my vindicator, He holds the scales of injustice.

We can learn a lot about injustice and forgiveness from the life of Jesus. Jesus taught us to love our enemies; he understood the profound truth that love conquers all. The life of Jesus was a mission of love and His death was no exception. Throughout His final hours on earth His love was pushed beyond human comprehension. He was suffering in a way that we cannot begin to even partially understand; yet all the while he remained in love with his accusers … The perfect example of what true forgiveness looks like. I can't imagine the restraint of Jesus as the guards blindfolded him and were mocking and beating him. A crown of thorns pierced his forehead and the fierce crowd shouting, "Crucify him," but the whole time forgiveness was on his mind. Nailed to a cross, nearing death, our Saviour continued to love His enemies and with mercy in His heart he cried "Father, forgive them, for they do not know what they do" (Luke 23:34, NKJV).

According to Luke, in chapter 23:39, there were two criminals crucified either side of Jesus. One of His co-accused yelled abuse at Jesus, mocking Him "If You are the Christ, save Yourself and us" (NKJV). He was indeed the Christ. This truth became apparent to the other criminal as he sensed something in Jesus that moved him. Some would argue that he was moved by fear, knowing he wasn't to come down from the cross alive and in that moment he was repentant in such a way that at the very hour of his death, he cried a plea of mercy to the Son of God. He said "Lord, remember me when You come into Your kingdom." Jesus' response was the epitome of love and forgiveness. Though certainly undeserved, Jesus responded to the dying criminal with absolute understanding, acceptance, love, and compassion. Jesus said to him, "Assuredly, I say to you, today you will be with Me in Paradise" (Luke 23:42-43, NKJV). On my best days, my most "perfect Christian days," I struggle to fathom such a response, such a depth of love for His enemies, while He hung nailed to a cross. The crucifixion of Jesus Christ is an image which underscores forgiveness beyond measure.

The importance of forgiveness toward others is a matter which must be addressed if we are to experience peace, joy and happiness. Just as your spirit and soul will flourish when you offer forgiveness, so too your physical being will begin complete healing.

Jesus gave us many lessons on *offering* forgiveness toward others, but more importantly Jesus wants you to *receive* forgiveness. When the crucified criminal announced his faith in Jesus he was cleansed from all sin and accepted as a child of God. In the same way the gift of eternal life is conferred upon us when we come to Him and ask to *receive* forgiveness. When you come before Him and invite Him into your heart, just like the criminal on the cross, He will graciously receive you as His beloved child. Despite your past indiscretions you are a prized possession in the eyes of God. Through faith in Him you can experience the awesome grace and love of a Heavenly Father, a father that will calm your fearful heart and soothe your pain.

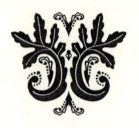

Chapter 29

Love on Purpose = Return to Joy

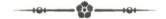

There are random moments throughout each day … a burst of laughter from my children, gazing out of the kitchen window and looking at the rainbow lorikeets dancing from branch to branch in the wattle trees, a saucepan of chai tea brewing on the stove top … when I feel the spirit of Joy flow through the caverns of my being. It is in this moment that I am grateful for the gift of life. I have come to realise that a life without Joy is a life that never reaches its full potential. If anything, the absence of Joy from one's life is like a fresh blossom devoid of water and sunlight. Before long, the blossom begins to wilt and lose its vibrant colour and eventually fades and dies, long before it reaches the beautiful, majestic flower it was created to be. Fullness of joy exists in God's presence (see Psalm 16:11). Joy is an expression of the Kingdom and a powerful healer for the body and mind. In his chapter, *Healing and the Kingdom* written within *The Essential Guide to Healing*, Bill Johnson summarises the value of joy: "Weeping is often an expression of repentance, but

176

laughter is an expression of joy. And what weeping is to repentance, laughter is to salvation. Solomon explains the physical body's response to joy when he states, "A joyful heart is good medicine" (Proverbs 17:22, NKJV). Joy has a healing effect on the body and mind. And as a kingdom manifestation, it is priceless" (Johnson and Clark, 125).

Perhaps you are in a place devoid of life, much like I was when my life was in the pit of depression. I want to encourage you, remind you and help you build the faith that you too can know that there is hope, and you will return to joy! If you will choose love, take your eyes off yourself and your problems and ask God, "Whom can I love today?" When you do this, your mind cannot be meditating on how bad you feel, but instead will be consumed with how you can be a blessing.

This morning I awoke feeling a little flat, hormonal and emotional, but as I do every morning, I asked God to "show me someone who needs love today." As I did this I felt joy begin to bubble up in my spirit. Instead of placing undue value on the natural realm of how you are feeling, lift up your eyes and get Heaven's perspective, partner with the Kingdom of God where it is not eating and drinking, but righteousness, peace and joy in the Holy Spirit (see Romans 14:17).

Righteousness, peace and joy are the manifestations of a life yielded to God. This is His plan for you. You see, the happiest people in this world are not the takers; the happiest people in this world are the givers! By choosing to think about giving/showing love to someone, you are harnessing the power of the Holy Spirit, the power of love. It is in this act that you increase the "feel good" chemicals in the brain, your heart starts to feel alive again and you feel a return to joy!

Jesus' life and death are the perfect representation of love leading to joy whereby He chose to love us by laying down His life for all mankind, He endured the cross and He returned to joy. In John 10:18, Jesus said of His life: *"No one takes it from Me, but I lay it down of Myself. I have power to lay it down, and I have power to take it again ..."* (NKJV). Here He is "choosing" to love for the joy that awaited Him. *"Looking unto Jesus, the author and finisher of our faith, who for the joy that was set before Him endured the cross, despising the shame, and has sat down at the right hand of the throne of God"* (Hebrews 12:2, NKJV). Choose today to "love on purpose" and watch as the spirit of Joy apprehends you.

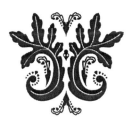

PART FIVE

FINAL THOUGHTS

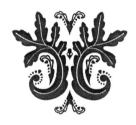

Chapter 30

Fearfully and Wonderfully Made

"You are the only you God made ... God made you and broke the mould." - Max Lucado

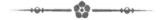

Now it's party time, time for a celebration! What are we celebrating? YOU my lovely, we are celebrating the FACT that you are fearfully and wonderfully made. God doesn't make junk, He makes everything glorious, one of His names is Wonderful. He made you and lives in you and that makes YOU Gloriously Wonderful or Wonderfully Glorious ... either way you look at it, you are pretty special.

As I write the close of this book, my smile is broad and my heart is full with the knowledge that the testimony of God's goodness in my life, His wonderful works, has filled both these pages and you, the reader, with hope and anticipation of living an astonishingly wonderful life, walking in the freedom, joy and unceasing love that He paid so great a price for us to have. Together, we can rejoice with the Psalmist and declare,

For it was you who formed my inward parts; you knit me together in my mother's womb. I praise you, for I am fearfully and wonderfully made. Wonderful are your works; that I know very well.

My frame was not hidden from you, when I was being made in secret, intricately woven in the depths of the earth.

Your eyes beheld my unformed substance. In your book were written all the days that were formed for me, when none of them as yet existed.

How weighty to me are your thoughts, O God! How vast is the sum of them!

I try to count them—they are more than the sand; I come to the end —I am still with you" (Psalm 139:13-18, NKJV).

Chapter 31

Call Back

It shall turn to you for a testimony – Luke 21:13

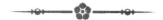

In the book of Revelation, John the Revelator writes, "The testimony of Jesus is the spirit of prophecy" (Revelation 19:10, NKJV). What this means to me is that what God has done in my life He will do again in your life and the lives of others. This has been the very inspiration for me to write "Beautiful, Courageous YOU," to share my testimony of being healed, delivered and completely set free from depression. To "call back," if you will, cheering you on, inspiring you and beckoning you into the place where peace and joy become your lifelong companions.

You may have heard it said when someone does a good deed you "pay it forward?" Paying it forward is a novel idea to change the world for the better; we can all manage that – right? In depression, I would have found it very difficult to get about and do good things for others … I simply had nothing left. No energy, no emotion, no inspiration – nothing. What I did have though was my life experience and as I began to heal from depression I found people, both men and women, who struggled with depression and who were naturally drawn to me for inspiration and encouragement. It is with this in mind that I wish to bring our journey as author and reader to a close by encouraging you, as you heal (and you will) to please remember those among us that are far behind in the healing journey and "call back." Help a friend along this stony track.

Mrs. Charles E. Cowman, a missionary in Japan and China, in 1925 penned these words with the notion in mind to "call back:"

> "Life is a steep climb, and it does the heart good to have somebody "call back" and cheerily beckon us on up the high hill. We are all climbers together, and we must help one another. This mountain climbing is serious business, but glorious. It takes strength and steady step to find the summits. The outlook widens with the altitude. If anyone among us has found anything worthwhile, we ought to "call back.""

With poetic splendour she continues ...

> "If you have gone a little way ahead of me, call back – 'Twill cheer my heart and help my feet along the stony track; And if, perchance, Faith's light is dim, because the oil is low, Your call will guide my lagging course as weerily I go.
>
> Call back, and tell me that He went with you into the storm; Call back, and say He kept you when the forests roots were torn; That, when the heavens thunder and the earthquake shook the hill, He bore you up and held you where the very air was still.
>
> Oh, friend call back, and tell me for I cannot see your face; They say it glows with triumph, and your feet bound in the

race; But there are mists between us and my spirit eyes are dim, And I cannot see the glory, though I long for word of Him.

But if you'll say He heard you when your prayer was but a cry, And if you'll say He saw you through the nights sin-darkened sky – If you have gone a little way ahead, oh, friend call back – 'Twill cheer my heart and help my feet along the stony track" (368).

A final thought from me is this: right now you may be the friend that requires a "call back." You might have found yourself in a place where your faith is dim and your prayer is but a cry. And yes, these may be the facts, however His Truth trumps your facts. The Lord's Truth is what His Word says about you. You are more than a conqueror through Christ Jesus, all thing do work together for your good, He has a great plan for your life. These promises are your Truth! This I know very well. That this too shall pass; for what is fact is temporal and what is Truth is eternal. All Glory and Honour to Jesus our Eternal King.

Chapter 32

Tired of Religion … I Want a Relationship with Jesus

Be strong, courageous, and firm; fear not nor be in terror before them, for it is the Lord your God Who goes with you; He will not fail you or forsake you (Deuteronomy 31:6, AMP). The Bible tells us to "fear not," "do not be afraid," "be strong and of good courage" many times over and over. God is calling us to live boldly and courageously in Him. You may not feel bold and courageous but the truth is, we are daughters of the King, and that fact allows us to be bold, confident and courageous even when we don't *feel* like it. Intimacy with Jesus is key to knowing who you are and who's you are. It is in this revelation of your identity that you will learn how to step out of fear and into the courage that comes with our inheritance as a beloved child of God.

If you're tired of religion, just going through the motions of an inherited set of rituals or working your way into favour with God through works-based Christianity … It's time to "Be Still" and know Him. There's nothing you can do to earn your way into Heaven, none is righteous, no not one, it's by His Grace alone that we are saved. You cannot do more to make the Lord love you. He loves you, because He loves you … Because that's what He is like. Come away for a little while with Him, lay aside your agenda, commit or perhaps re-commit yourself to your Heavenly Father and simply sit at His feet and rest in His perfect love for you.

God is not impressed with long-winded babble. The words you use in committing your life to God are not important. The Bible says that He knows the intentions of your heart. If the words don't come easy for you, this little prayer might help:

> Jesus, I want to know you intimately. I want you to come into my heart and be Lord of my life. Thank you for dying on the cross for my sin, so that I could be fully accepted by you. I surrender all that I am and commit my life to you. I ask that you do with my life as you will. Only you can give me the power to change and become the person you created me to be. Thank you for forgiving me and giving me eternal life with God. From this moment on may I bring you glory in all that I do. Amen.

If you sincerely asked Jesus into your life just now, then he has come into your life as he promised. You have begun your personal relationship with God. What follows is a lifelong journey of change and growth as you get to know God better through Bible reading, prayer and interaction with other Christians.

SHARE YOUR STORIES
OF BEAUTY AND COURAGE

Perhaps you have come to the end of this book and feel inspired from my story and hopeful with the general information shared on healing for the spirit, soul and body. Much like I used to respond when hearing a testimony or reading a powerful story of overcoming adversity, you might be thinking, "Well, that's great for Lauralee, praise God that she is well, but He probably won't do that for me!"

Now it is your chance to inspire or be inspired. I am inviting all beautiful, courageous women … that means ALL of you, to share your stories. You embody beauty and courage in your own uniquely magnificent way. Yes this is TRUE, this is YOU and in the words of Dr. Seuss "Today you are You, that is truer than true. There is no one alive who is Youer than you." Oh how I would love to pull up a chair with you, recline, and listen as you share your story, for sure we'd laugh and cry together, but above all we could encourage one another through life's valleys and celebrate upon life's mountaintops. It's for this reason that I have opened the *Beauty and Courage* network. A place where you can come and meet with other women, share your stories of overcoming, inspire others that are on the healing journey, share images of beauty and courage and enjoy community with one another via the website www.beautfulcourageousyou.com. Finally, if you have a testimony of how the content in this book has helped you, I would be delighted to hear about it!

Blessings, Lauralee x

BIBLIOGRAPHY

Beckham, Dr. Ed. "Stress, Cortisol And Depression." *drbeckham.blogspot.com.au.* Dr. Ed Beckham, 2010. Web. 7 June 2013.

Bhattacharya SK, et al. "Anxiolytic-Antidepressant Activity Of Withania Somnifera Glycowithanolides: An Experimental Study. - Pubmed - NCBI." *PubMed.gov.* <u>National Center for Biotechnology Information, U.S. National Library of Medicine</u>, 2000. Web. 20 Aug. 2015.

Breus, Michael J. "Better Sleep Found By Exercising On A Regular Basis." *Psychology Today.* Psychology Today, 2013. Web. 5 Feb. 2014.

Chan, F. and Yankoski, D. *Crazy Love.* Colorado Springs, Colo.: David C. Cook, 2008. Print.

Conner, Bobby. "Bobby Conner: How To Maintain A Tranquil Soul." *Elijahlist.com.* The Elijah List, 2012. Web. 28 Aug. 2015.

Cowman, Mrs Charles E. *Streams In The Desert.* Grand Rapids, Mich.: Zondervan, 1996. Print.

Craft, L.L. and Perna, F.M. "The Benefits Of Exercise For The Clinically Depressed." *Primary Care Companion to The Journal of Clinical Psychiatry* 6.3 (2004): 104. Web. 8 Aug. 2015.

"Elisabeth Kübler-Ross Foundation." *ekrfoundation.org.* Elisabeth Kübler-Ross Foundation, 2015. Web. 6 June 2015.

Gass, Bob. "Courage (2)." *thewordfortoday.com.au.* Vision Christian Media, 2012. Web. 3 Sept. 2015.

Gass, Bob. "When You Can't Understand, Trust God." *thewordfortoday. com.au.* Vision Christian Media, 2012. Web. 26 Aug. 2015.

Gass, B. and Gass, D. "Satan Is Defeated (4)." *thewordfortoday.com.au.* Vision Christian Media, 2012. Web. 7 Jan. 2014.

Giglio, Louie. *The Air I Breathe.* Sisters, Ore.: Multnomah Publishers, 2003. Print.

"Gill's Exposition Proverbs 4." *biblehub.com.* Bible Hub. n.d. Web. 7 Aug. 2015.

"Helen Keller | The Story Of My Life | TO REV. PHILLIPS BROOKS." *Afb.org.* American Foundation for the Blind, 2015. Web. 26 Aug. 2015.

Holford, Patrick. "The Low GL Diet Bible - Patrick Holford Books." *Patrickholford.com.* Natural Wellbeing Limited, 2015. Web. 10 Aug. 2015.

"Home." *foodforthebrain.org.* Food for the Brain, 2012. Web. 10 Aug. 2015.

Jacka FN, et al. "Association Of Western And Traditional Diets With Depression And Anxiety In Women. - Pubmed - NCBI." *Ncbi. nlm.nih.gov.* National Center for Biotechnology Information, U.S. National Library of Medicine, 2010. Web. 1 June 2014.

Jacobsen, Wayne. *He Loves Me!* Newbury Park, Calif.: Windblown Media, 2007. Print.

Johnson, B, and Clark, R. *The Essential Guide To Healing*. Grand Rapids, Mich.: Chosen, 2011. Print.

Keller, Timothy. *The Reason For God*. Grand Rapids, Mich.: Zondervan, 2010. Print.

Lawlor, D.A. and Hopker, S.W. "The Effectiveness Of Exercise As An Intervention In The Management Of Depression: Systematic Review And Meta-Regression Analysis Of Randomised Controlled Trials." *BMJ : British Medical Journal* 322.7289 (2001): 763. Web. 8 Aug. 2015.

Leaf, Caroline. *Who Switched Off My Brain?* Thomas Nelson, 2009. Print.

"Lexicon :: Strong's H1350 - Ga'al." *blueletterbible.org*. Blue Letter Bible, 2015. Web. 28 Aug. 2015.

"Lord, I Believe; Help My Unbelief." *dailyexegesis.blogspot.com.au*. Daily Exegesis, 24 Mar. 2012. Web. 3 Aug. 2014.

Lucado, Max. *Outlive Your Life*. Nashville, Tenn.: Thomas Nelson, 2010. Print.

MacArthur, John. *Alone With God*. Wheaton, Ill.: Victor Books, 1995. Print

Mattson, M. and Wan, R. "Beneficial Effects Of Intermittent Fasting And Caloric Restriction On The Cardiovascular And Cerebrovascular Systems. - Pubmed - NCBI". *Ncbi.nlm.nih.gov*. National Center for Biotechnology Information, U.S. National Library of Medicine, 2005. Web. 2 Apr. 2013.

McMillen, Matt. "Benefits Of Exercise To Help With Depression." *WebMD*. WebMD, 2010. Web. 2 Apr. 2013.

Mercyme."The Hurt & The Healer - Official Music Video." Online video clip. *YouTube*. YouTube, 21 May. 2012. Web. 26 Aug. 2015.

Meyer, Joyce. *Battlefield Of The Mind*. New York, N.Y.: Warner, 2002. Print.

Meyer, Joyce. *Never Give Up!* New York: Faith Words, 2008. Print.

Meyer, Joyce. *The Everyday Life Bible*. New York: Warner Faith, 2006. Print.

"Nelson Mandela Biography: Life For Freedom." Online video clip. *YouTube*. IgeoNews, 17 Oct. 2013. Web. 26 Aug. 2015.

"Oil Garden Aromatherapy Australia - FAQ." *oilgarden.com.au*. Heritage Brands Pty Ltd, 2013. Web. 10 Aug. 2015.

"*Omega-3 And Mood Disorders*. 1st ed." Randwick NSW: The Black Dog Institute, 2012. Web. 8 Aug. 2015.

Popa, T.A., and Ladea, M. "Nutrition And Depression At The Forefront Of Progress." *Journal of Medicine and Life* 5.4 (2012). University Press. Web. 8 Aug. 2015.

Quinn, B., Yancey, P., and Moon, S. *What's So Amazing About Grace?* Grand Rapids, Mich.: Zondervan, 2000. Print.

Roth, Sid. "*Sid Roth Welcomes Dr. Caroline Leaf.*" Online video clip. *YouTube*. Sid Roth's It's Supernatural, 2010. Web. 7 Feb. 2011.

"Spiritual Thirst." *Biblecentre.com*. Bible Center, 2015. Web. 3 Sept. 2015.

Spurgeon, Charles H. *Why Is Faith So Feeble?* 1st ed. Newington: Spurgeon Gems. Web. 26 Aug. 2015.

"Touch Research Institute." *www6.miami.edu*. Ubniversity of Miami, n.d. Web. 10 Aug. 2015.

Van Schie, Jason. "An Hour Before Midnight Is Worth Two After." *Sleephealthfoundation.org.au*. Sleep Health Foundation, n.d. Web. 5 Feb. 2014.

Vujicic, Nick. "Life Without Limits Quotes." *Goodreads.com*. Goodreads Inc., 2015. Web. 12 January 2015

Warren, Rick. "Daily Hope With Rick Warren; Quit Trying to Please Everybody." *Rickwarren.org*. Rick Warren, 2014. Web. 21 May 2014.

Warren, Rick. "Daily Hope With Rick Warren; Why Worry?" *Rickwarren.org*. Rick Warren, 2014. Web. 21 May 2014.

Watts, Kristi. "Nick Vujicic: Life Without Limbs < Guests On The 700 Club." *cbn.com*. The Christian Broadcasting Network, Inc., 2015. Web. 28 Aug. 2015.

"What Causes Depression" *beyondblue.org.au*. Beyond Blue Ltd., 2014. Web. 8 Aug. 2015.

"What Causes Depression? - Harvard Health." *Harvard Health*. Harvard Publications, 2015. Web. 8 Aug. 2015.

"What Is Toxic Thinking Anyway?" *ccsng.com*. CCSNG. n.d. Web. 7 Aug. 2015.

Wiersbe, Warren W. *The Wiersbe Bible Commentary*. Colorado Springs: David C Cook, 2007. Print.

BIBLE VERSIONS USED

Meyer, Joyce. *The Everyday Life Bible*. New York: Warner Faith, 2006. Print.

Peterson, Eugene H. *The Message*. Colorado Springs, CO: NavPress, 2004. Print.

Radmacher, E.D., Allen, R.B. and House, H.W. *NKJV Study Bible*. Nashville: Thomas Nelson, 2007. Print.

CPSIA information can be obtained
at www.ICGtesting.com
Printed in the USA
LVOW12s1831241117
557401LV00002B/123/P

9 780646 966205